Essential
KETO
BREAD

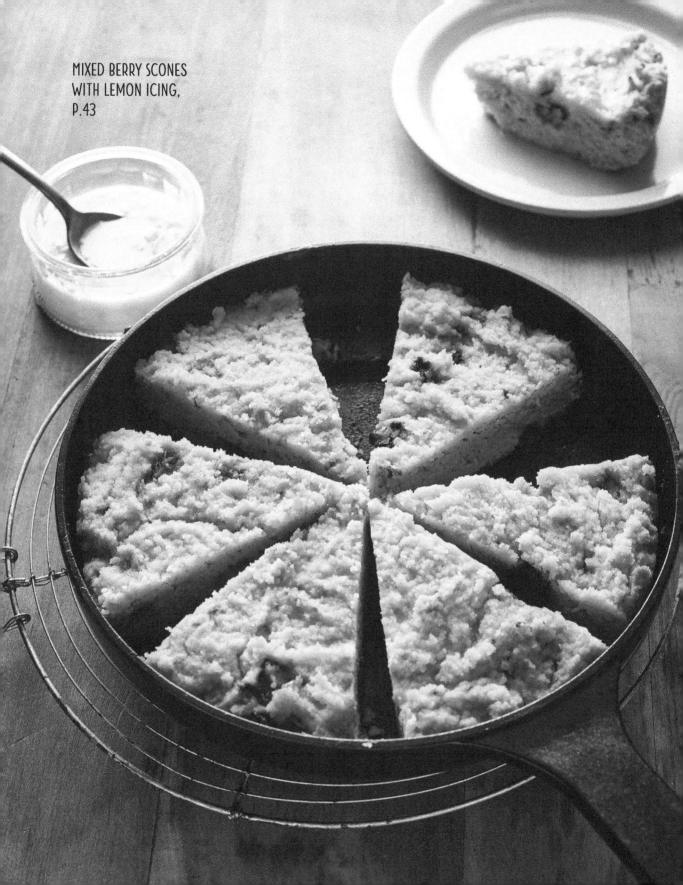

MIXED BERRY SCONES
WITH LEMON ICING,
P.43

Essential
KETO
BREAD

SWEET AND SAVORY BAKED GOODS
TO SATISFY ANY CRAVING

HILDA SOLARES

PHOTOGRAPHY BY EMULSION STUDIO

ROCKRIDGE
PRESS

Interior and Cover Designer: Peatra Jariva
Editor: Ada Fung
Production Editor: Kurt Shulenberger
Photography © 2019 Emulsion Studio
Author photo courtesy of © Hilda Solares

ISBN: Print 978-1-64152-893-1 | eBook 978-1-64152-894-8

R0

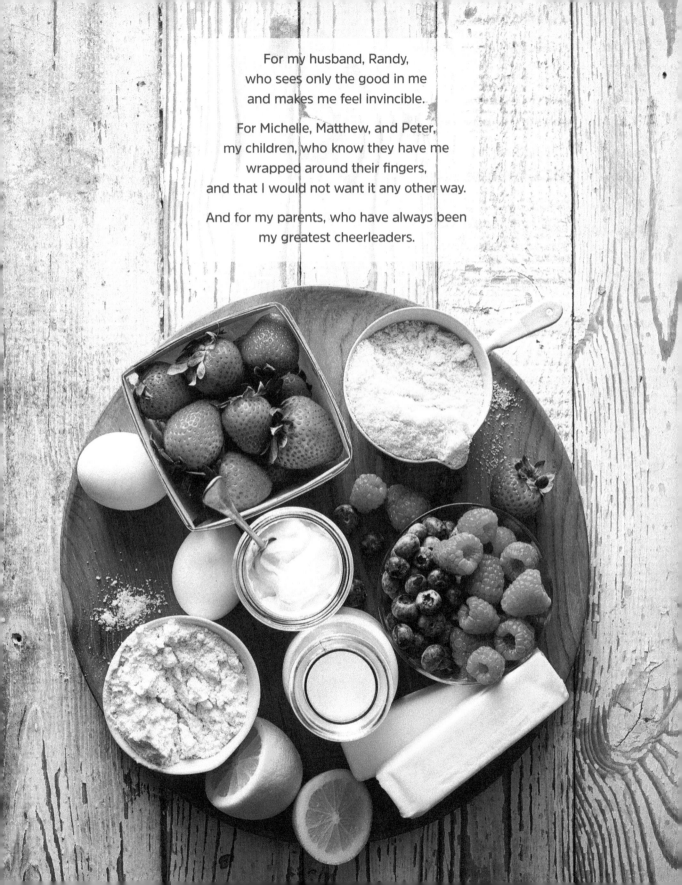

For my husband, Randy,
who sees only the good in me
and makes me feel invincible.

For Michelle, Matthew, and Peter,
my children, who know they have me
wrapped around their fingers,
and that I would not want it any other way.

And for my parents, who have always been
my greatest cheerleaders.

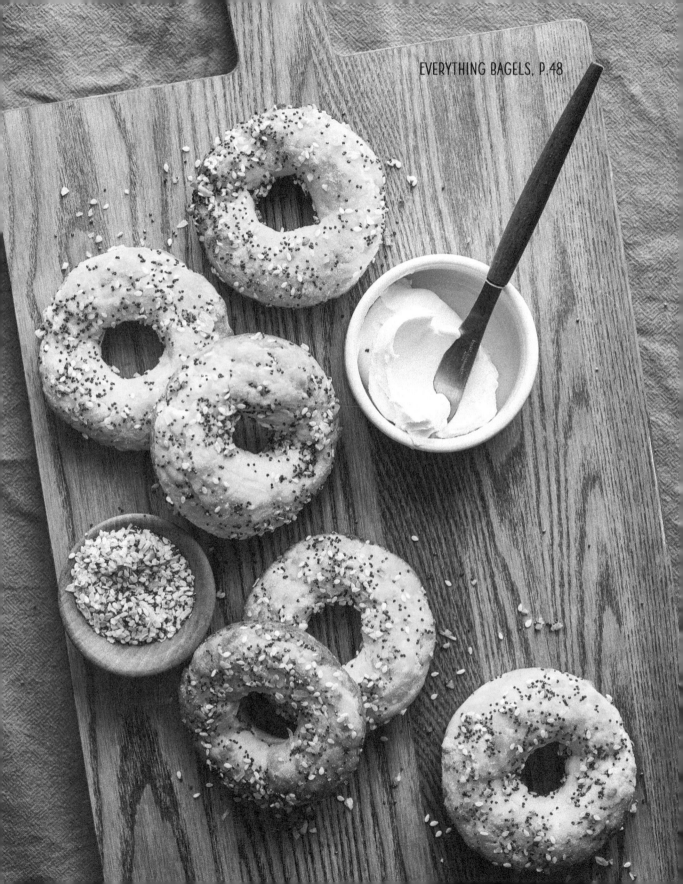

EVERYTHING BAGELS, P.48

CONTENTS

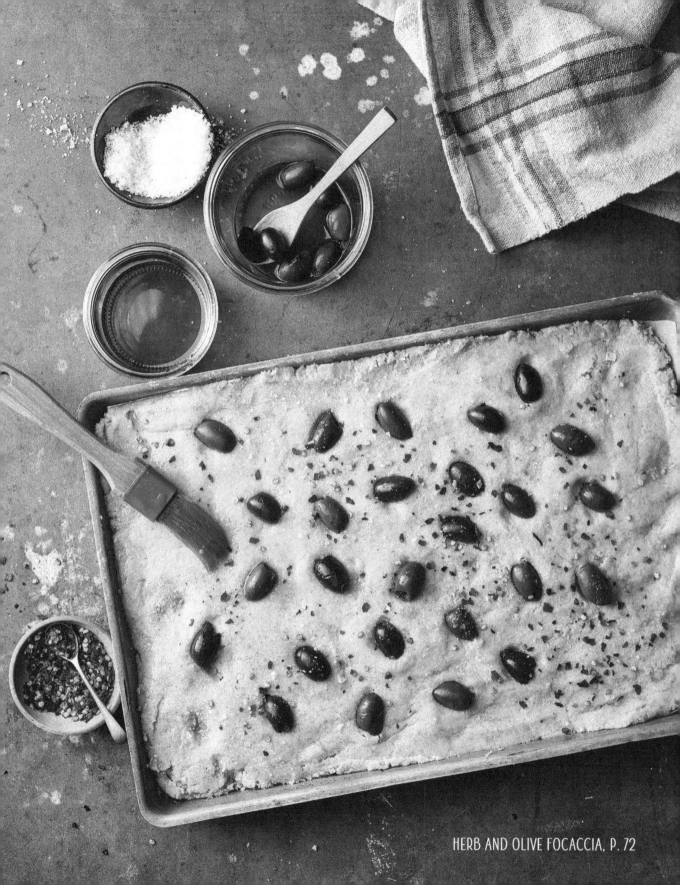

HERB AND OLIVE FOCACCIA, P. 72

INTRODUCTION

What should have destroyed me, today serves to inspire. When I was diagnosed with Guillain-Barré syndrome and fibromyalgia in 2001, it felt like a life sentence of pain and weakness. Thankfully, it wasn't.

In 2006, after years of battling symptoms and having them only get worse, I made the difficult decision to leave my lifelong academic career. Uncertain of my future, I cried out to God for an answer. His response was simple: Remove sugar and grains from my diet. I obeyed, and it was then that I inadvertently tapped into the benefits of the keto diet.

For two solid years, I was committed to the diet, and my health dramatically improved. But my intense carb cravings got the best of me. And so I rationalized that because I was better, there would be no harm in returning to my old eating patterns. Unfortunately, that decision caused my health to spin out of control. And at my worst, I needed a walker and was on a morphine patch for almost a year.

Finally, at the end of 2013, I saw the error of my ways and realized that abstaining from sugar and grains was the only way for me to be healthy.

In January 2014, my husband, Randy, and I decided to make this way of eating a lifestyle. I began to research everything I could about the keto diet. What I learned inspired me to experiment with creating keto-friendly dishes. My first attempts caused a lot of frustration, but I was determined to make the lifestyle work.

The transformation we experienced was dramatic. Randy lost more than 80 pounds and reversed his diabetes. I regained strength and got rid of the fatigue that had plagued me for years.

Intrigued by our results, family and friends wanted to learn what we were doing. Our pastors gave us the green light to form a community group in which we have since supported others who want similar results. Our blog FitToServeGroup.com became the vehicle for us to share our journey and a place to post my low-carb keto recipes for others to enjoy.

Knowing firsthand the importance of staying committed is why I am passionate about creating recipes that make the keto lifestyle more accessible. Today, when I experience carb cravings, I use it as an opportunity to create new recipes.

I was inspired to write this keto baking book to be able to offer a resource that would make it easier to address carb cravings with recipes that are not only delicious but also simple to make. I hope it helps keep you on your path to good health and a good life.

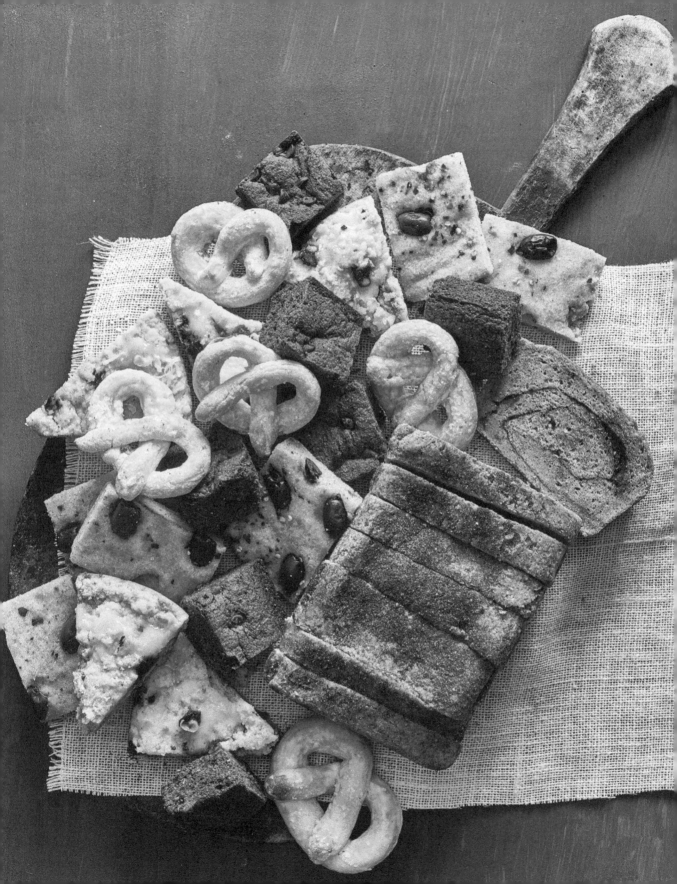

CHAPTER 1

HAVE YOUR CAKE
AND KETO, TOO

Anyone who's ever attempted the keto diet will tell you that baked goods are at the top of the list of items they miss. Succumbing to the temptation of traditional bread, muffins, cakes, and cookies is why people quit the diet before seeing any of its benefits. If giving up your favorite carbs seems like an impossible feat, I am here to show you how you can experience the benefits of keto and still have cake, too.

WHY BAKE KETO BREADS?

I understand why the prospect of giving up bread or carb-heavy dishes seems impossible—it's hard to ignore their strong pull. Carb cravings can drive anyone to throw in the towel before seeing any lasting results. Learning how to bake keto bread is definitely worth your time.

Although this cookbook is full of bread recipes like loaves and rolls, it also includes pancakes, muffins, cakes, bagels, pizza, cookies, and more. Making these crave-worthy recipes will reward you with the ability to stick to the ketogenic diet long-term. You will find delicious and exciting ways to silence your carb cravings and stay satisfied.

A KETO REFRESHER

Without a doubt, the keto diet has become a hot trend. But what is behind its enormous popularity? Well, the results speak for themselves, with countless testimonials backing up this way of eating. People are finding that the keto diet is an effective way to lose weight, control hunger, silence cravings, improve cognition, and even help prevent or alleviate symptoms of chronic diseases.

The goal of the keto diet is to get the body into a state of therapeutic ketosis. What is ketosis, and why is it desirable? I like to think of ketosis as a better fuel source for the body. Our bodies are designed to run on either glucose (sugar) or ketones (fat). In the absence of glucose, the body looks for an alternative fuel source and turns to fatty acids and fat stores to provide the energy it needs.

When your body transitions into ketosis, it burns fat for fuel (instead of sugar) by creating ketones. While in ketosis, a person has elevated ketone levels, typically above 0.5 mmol/L. Here is where the magic happens, because ketosis gives you more sustainable energy. Rather than your energy constantly dipping, you now have a vast resource.

Your liver begins to break down the fat and releases ketones to be used by your brain and other organs. Fat-burning begins, and stored fat starts to melt away. While on a keto diet, fat is burned more effectively, which is the number one reason people are turning to the keto diet for fat loss.

However, the benefits of ketosis do not end there. Ketones are the fuel our brains seem to prefer. And that explains why people on the keto diet experience a state of hyperfocus and improved cognitive function.

The keto diet contains between 20 and 50 grams of net carbs per day; net carbs are the total number of carbs minus fiber. That means only 5 to 10 percent of total daily calories come from carbohydrates. What's the difference between a low-carb diet and a keto diet? Although the two are similar, the main difference is that the keto diet is higher in fat and allows for a range of dietary fats, which make up anywhere from 70 to 80 percent of total daily calories. So, you can say it is a diet that has four times more fat than carbs and protein.

MANAGING MACRONUTRIENTS

Whether or not you see the benefits of a keto diet will hinge on how well you manage your macronutrients (also known as macros): fat, proteins, and carbohydrates. While it is tempting to say that a keto diet is just a diet that's 70 percent fat, 25 percent protein, and 5 percent carbohydrate, to do so would be an oversimplification.

Unfortunately, just counting macros does not take into account individual differences, such as overall health, physical activity, and calorie intake. There are some significant differences between a bodybuilder doing a keto diet and an average person who just wants to lose some weight. To effectively do the keto diet, you will have to personalize your macros to your own unique circumstances. Many free keto calculators can assist you in determining your macros, such as the one from Perfect Keto (see Resources, page 132). Once you know your ideal macro numbers—that is, the percentage of fat, protein, and carbohydrate in your daily diet—you can plan your meals effectively.

One of the things I love about the keto diet is having the flexibility to balance your macros in such a way that you can decide to splurge on a more substantial meal, say at dinner, by planning a smaller breakfast or lunch. Or you can choose to divide your macros evenly throughout the day.

HIGH FAT

We've already established that the keto diet is pretty high in fats. Keep in mind that the quality of the fat matters. Aim to include natural forms of both saturated and unsaturated fats. Examples of natural saturated fats include animal-based fats such as lard, dairy-based fats such as butter, and coconut-based fats such as coconut oil. All of these become solid at room temperature. Unsaturated fats are liquid at room temperature and are typically vegetable-based. These include olive oil, avocado oil, and nut oils. The fats to avoid are trans fats, which are manufactured and are found primarily in processed foods and fast food.

MODERATE PROTEIN

While protein plays a vital role in your diet and supplies the building blocks for body tissue, muscles, and hormone signaling, protein consumption is moderate on a keto diet because a higher intake of protein can make it challenging to get into ketosis.

The amount of protein that's right for you is related to your activity level. Protein macros can range between 15 and 30 percent of total calories. Stay at the lower range if you're not as active and at the higher range if you're quite active.

LOW CARBOHYDRATE

Crucial to the success of the keto diet is that carbohydrate levels be kept low to prevent spikes in blood glucose and insulin, which keep you from entering ketosis.

On a keto diet, evidence supports focusing on net carbs rather than total carbs. Net carbs are the carbs your body processes and then uses for energy; you calculate it by subtracting fiber and also some sugar alcohols from the total number of carbs. Although fiber is considered a carbohydrate, most of the fiber you eat is eliminated rather than absorbed by the body. This is why most people on a keto diet track net carbs instead of total carbs.

THE DEAL WITH KETO BAKING

Keto baking can be intimidating if you are used to conventional flour recipes. Unfortunately, it is not just a matter of swapping in low-carb ingredients for high-carb ones; they do not bake the same way. While it is possible to create delicious keto baked goods, they will not, however, be 100 percent the same as high-carb ones. It's a small trade-off for having options that will enable you to stick with the diet.

The good news is that keto baking can take less time. For example, you will not have to proof your bread the same way you would with gluten-based recipes that use yeast as a starter. Another benefit is that keto baking uses nutrition-packed ingredients like real butter, cream, nut flours, and high-fiber options like coconut flour and flax meal. These are superior to white all-purpose flour and sugar, both of which are just empty calories.

The lack of gluten in keto breads means the texture will be different. Achieving a chewy or crispy texture is trickier and requires you to use specific techniques or ingredients to come close to conventional counterparts. Keto breads are also a bit denser compared to standard ones, and it is why they usually call for more leavening agents.

BALANCING YOUR MACROS WITH KETO BREADS

Once you know your ideal macros, incorporating recipes like Cream Cheese Pound Cake (page 123) into your diet becomes easier. By lowering your servings or changing an allocated meal for the day, you can enjoy a treat but still keep to your daily macros. For example, if you make one of your meals a green leafy salad topped with a moderate amount of fish or meat, you will have enough macros left over to have some cookies at the end of the day.

INGREDIENTS THAT MAKE A DIFFERENCE

The following ingredients are used in keto baking because they help add stability and structure—important considerations when you are baking without gluten.

Egg whites: When exposed to heat, egg whites thicken and solidify. In keto baking, you will see that eggs play a significant role. They help bind ingredients in the absence of gluten and ensure that the baked goods, like Raspberry-Lemon Pound Cake (page 126), have the stability they need and do not fall apart.

Cream of tartar: Cream of tartar is potassium bitartrate, the acidic byproduct of grape fermentation. A pinch of it can help stabilize egg whites when they are whipped before adding them to a recipe. It strengthens the foam and prevents the egg from collapsing too quickly. Cream of tartar can also add a bit of acidity to enhance a recipe like Snickerdoodle Bars (page 102).

Cream cheese: Cream cheese is used to help add stability and moisture to keto baked goods. It can play a role in improving the structure of Everything Bagels (page 48) and Lemon Cookies (page 93).

Gelatin: Adding a little unflavored gelatin powder can give some elasticity to your final baked goods. Gelatin can also act as a great thickener and binder in keto desserts like Chocolate Chunk Cookies (page 95). Gelatin is derived from the collagen of animals, and I recommend gelatin from grass-fed animals, such as the Vital Protein brand. But Great Lakes and Knox will work, as well.

TIPS FOR KETO BAKING SUCCESS

I like to share simple keto recipes. I believe you can get consistent results without complicated steps or hard-to-find ingredients. Keeping that in mind, here are some tips that will ensure your success.

USE HIGH-QUALITY INGREDIENTS

The quality of your ingredients plays a significant role in how your baked goods turn out. It's essential to use quality brands you know you can count on because they have a proven track record. For example, nut flours tend to go rancid quickly, and if a nut flour is made in a facility that does not have high demand, it is possible the flour won't be as fresh. This, in turn, will produce a baked good that can have an off taste.

I also recommend whenever possible to use butter from grass-fed cows. This is because it has five times more CLA, the fatty acid that can promote fat loss, than regular butter and is much higher in omega-3 fatty acids and vitamin K_2. Grass-fed also translates to superior flavor. That being said, you can still use regular butter and get good results with keto baking.

MEASURE ACCURATELY

When it comes to measuring ingredients, accuracy is vital in all types of baking. While a digital scale is most precise, many people don't know how to use one and can be intimidated. I've found that I can still get stellar results using standard measuring cups and spoons.

What's most important when measuring your ingredients, especially with non-wheat flours, is to not pack the flour in too tightly. To avoid this, spoon the ingredients into the measuring cup instead of using the cup to scoop them up. Doing this will give you better, more consistent results.

SIFTING MAKES A DIFFERENCE

Using a sifter may seem like an unnecessary step, especially when alternative flours are labeled as finely milled. However, it can make a significant difference, just as it does in non-keto baking. Sifting eliminates any coarse pieces of nuts, which can adversely affect the texture of your baked goods. This extra step is necessary when working with almond and hazelnut flours, as they are heavy flours and are more prone to having clumps and larger pieces. When using the recipes in this book, I recommend that you first measure and then sift for the best results, unless otherwise stated in the recipe.

CONTENTS

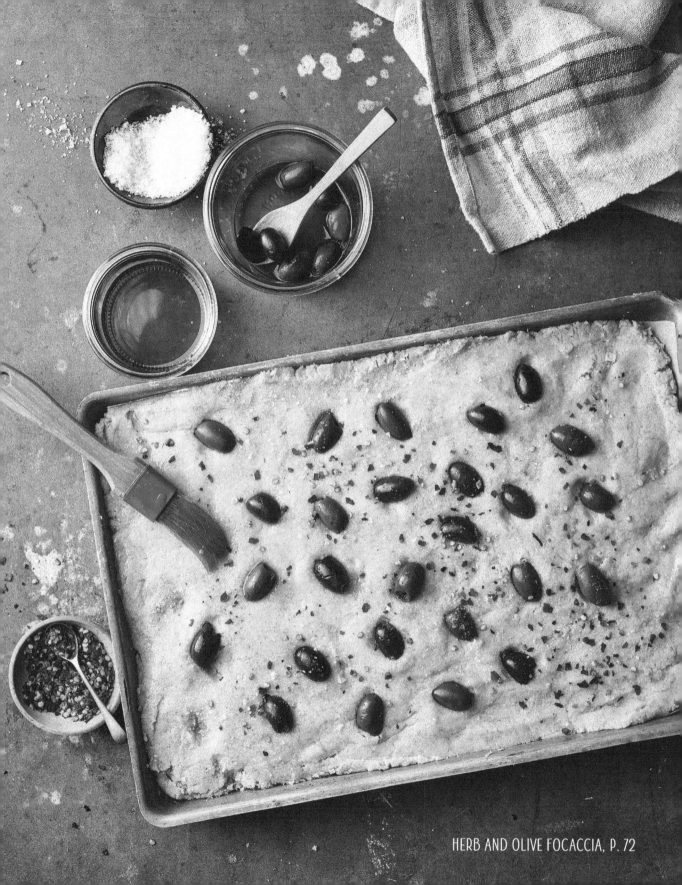

HERB AND OLIVE FOCACCIA, P. 72

MAKE KNOWLEDGEABLE SUBSTITUTIONS

There will be times when substitutions are necessary because you don't have something on hand, can't eat something, or just don't like a particular ingredient. It is essential to understand, though, that not all ingredients are interchangeable.

Alternative Flours

You can substitute hazelnut flour or pecan flour for almond meal, but not for blanched almond flour, which has a more delicate texture because it is processed without almond skins.

Coconut flour stands alone and can never be equally substituted for any nut flour because it is a much thirstier flour and does not have the same amount of moisture as nut flours. Recipes that use coconut flour have taken into consideration the need for additional moisture. The integrity of the recipe will be completely compromised if you attempt to substitute coconut flour for any other ingredient.

Fats

Some fats can be swapped successfully, but that's not always the case. A successful example is when a recipe calls for melted butter: You can substitute the same amount of melted coconut oil. The important thing to remember is that you can substitute liquid for liquid or solid for solid. Where you will run into issues is if you are trying to swap a solid, such as room-temperature butter, for a liquid, such as melted coconut oil.

Zero-Calorie Sweeteners

Granulated erythritol brands such as Lakanto or Swerve or xylitol brands such as NOW Foods (both are natural sugar alcohols) can be substituted in equal amounts for granulated white sugar. Pyure, an erythritol-stevia blend, is significantly sweeter, so you will need to use about half as much. Stevia-based sweeteners can be bitter, and they do not work well in chocolate recipes because the chocolate intensifies the aftertaste.

When you need a brown sugar alternative, Lakanto, Swerve, and Sukrin brands will give you comparable results. If a recipe calls for a confectioners' sugar substitute, Lakanto and Swerve have great options. You can also grind any of your granulated sweeteners in a dry blender until powdered. Keep in mind that when they are finely ground, the sweetness intensifies, so use them sparingly.

STORE KETO BREADS PROPERLY

The fact that these recipes generally use a higher amount of fat and dairy than wheat-flour breads means their shelf life is considerably shorter. You will find storage instructions with each recipe. But in general, I recommend double wrapping your baked goods in either plastic wrap or wax paper, then aluminum foil. Alternatively, you can store them in sealed airtight containers. Stored this way, they generally can be refrigerated for up to five days. If you plan to freeze something, wrap it as described, then place your bread in either a freezer bag or a freezer-safe container.

TROUBLESHOOTING KETO BAKING

These are common questions that I frequently hear from people who are learning keto baking. This will help address any concerns you may encounter.

Q. Why didn't my keto baked cake or loaf rise?

There can be several reasons, but in most cases, it's a leavening issue. Make sure your baking powder hasn't expired. Baking powder needs to be stored in a cool and dry place. If you store it in an area that has a lot of humidity and heat, your baking powder could expire sooner—which may be why the baked good has not risen properly.

Also, check to make sure you didn't use baking soda instead of baking powder—a common mistake! Baking soda needs an acid to activate, and if the recipe doesn't take this into consideration, your cake or bread will not rise properly.

Check your yeast's expiration date. Even if the yeast hasn't expired, it's a good idea to test it before using it in a recipe by blooming it. Add a teaspoon of sugar or inulin fiber to a little bit of lukewarm water. Sprinkle the yeast over the mix. If the yeast does not foam and then bubble, then it has probably expired.

Q. My dough keeps sticking to my hands, and it's hard to work with. Help!

Using alternative flours will mean some doughs will be sticky and hard to work with. The best way to address this is to keep your hands and your spatula wet while handling the dough. Keep a small bowl of water next to you while you are working, to make things easier.

Q. Why does my keto bread crumble and fall apart?

Did you use the number of eggs called for in the recipe? If you reduce the quantity, the dough may not bind properly. Also, if you omit the flaxseed or psyllium husk powder, the structure of your bread will be affected, as those serve as binders in the recipe. Make sure you're also letting your baked goods cool completely before handling; if not, they will likely crumble.

Q. My bread turned purple, what happened?

Bread may turn a shade of purple when using psyllium husk powder. Some brands have better results than others, but even if your bread has a purple tinge, it is safe to eat, and the color does not affect the taste or consistency of the product. I recommend using the NOW Foods brand, as it has yet to turn my bread purple.

Q. Why did my bread turn out dense and grainy?

This is not uncommon in recipes that use a lot of nut flour because nut flours are inherently heavier than traditional wheat flours. To avoid this, always measure and then sift your nut flours before adding them to the recipe. Sifting the flour will help your bread have a lighter texture and will remove any bits and pieces of coarse nuts in the mixture that can weigh it down.

HOW TO USE THIS BOOK

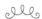

The goal of this keto bread book is to make the keto diet sustainable. By giving you delicious low-carb options, carb cravings will be kept to a minimum, and you will see lasting results. Deciding which recipes to include in this book required careful consideration. I wanted them to be easy to make, but I also wanted them to be as close as to their high-carb counterparts as possible.

It is important to note that not every recipe listed will meet the strict macro ideal of 70-25-5 (70 percent fats, 25 percent protein, 5 percent carbs). You can, however, still enjoy these keto baked goods by balancing the rest of your meals for the day. Although careful planning is necessary, these recipes will always be much lower in net carbs than what you typically find in other baking books, and they will include only strictly keto-friendly ingredients.

COUNTING CARBS

The recipes in this book will give you the net carbs in grams per serving of each dish, and provide the carb macro percentages.

The recipes that use yeast call for a small amount of sugar to proof the yeast. It's important to note that in the proofing process, the yeast feeds on the sugar and releases carbon dioxide gas. During this fermentation process, the sugar is used up, so it doesn't count toward net carbs either. However, if you are uncomfortable with adding any amount of sugar, you can use inulin fiber instead, with similar results (see page 17 for more on inulin).

RECIPE TIPS

To make these recipes extra easy to use, I have included a list of how many mixing bowls, appliances, and cooking vessels you will need to make each one. I also offer tips at the end of many recipes.

Keep in Mind: This tip offers advice to help increase the success of your final product and ensure consistency.

Ingredient Tip: This tip will assist you in selecting ingredients and understanding how to work with them.

Variation Tip: Some recipes will include a variation tip for adding or changing ingredients, such as add-ins or toppings.

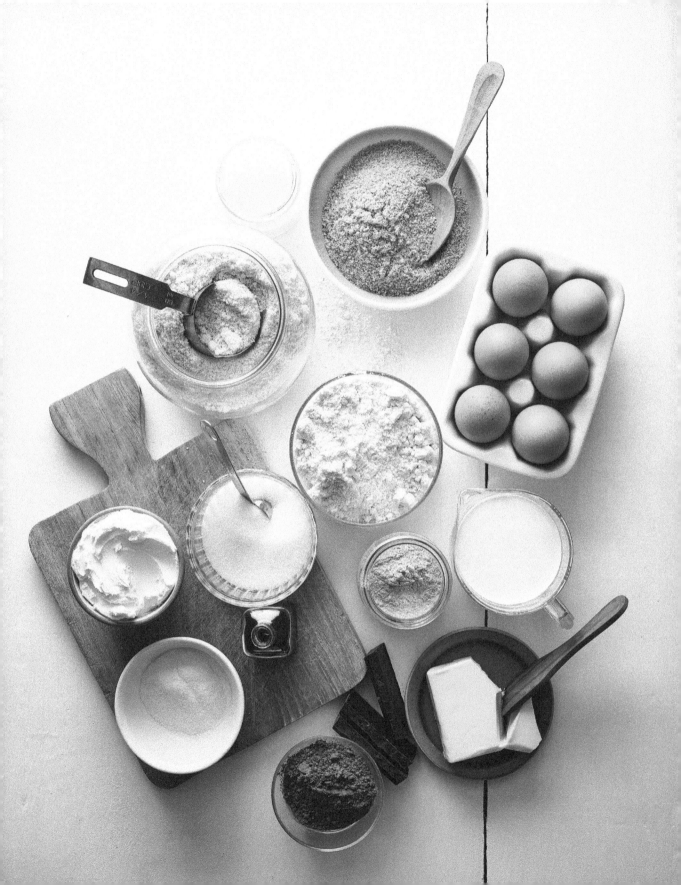

CHAPTER 2

THE KETO BAKER'S KITCHEN

Knowing exactly what ingredients and equipment you'll need for the recipes in this book will make your keto baking journey much easier because quality tools and ingredients will help ensure delicious, consistent results. In this chapter, I provide a rundown of the primary ingredients involved in keto baking, as well as a list of the necessary equipment to make the tasty and satisfying baked goods in this book. Once you've read this chapter and purchased what you need, go forth and bake!

THE KETO BAKER'S PANTRY

A properly stocked pantry is essential to help you succeed at keto baking. In this section, I've listed some of the ingredients you should keep stocked in your pantry to make these delicious recipes, including some of my preferred brands, so you know you're baking with tried and trusted ingredients.

KETO-FRIENDLY FLOURS

Low-carb flours tend to spoil quickly, so be sure to store them in airtight containers, and don't keep them too long. Many people keep nut flours in the refrigerator.

Almond Flour

Almond flour is made from blanched, skinned almonds that are finely ground into flour. It is a gluten-free nut flour with a mild, sweet, nutty aroma, which shines through in baked goods. The texture of finely milled almond flour comes closest to traditional wheat flour, which is why it's a popular choice in keto baking. It can be used exclusively in recipes, like my Cream Cheese Pound Cake (page 123), or in combination with other alternative flours. However, the number of carbohydrates can vary significantly between brands, so do look at the nutritional information and compare across brands before purchasing. My favorite brands are Bob's Red Mill and Anthony's Goods, which can be found online and in most national grocery stores.

Almond Meal

Almond meal, although similar to almond flour, is coarser because the skins are generally not removed. It works well in "corn bread" recipes, like my Southern Sweet Corn Bread (page 88), since the texture is similar to ground cornmeal. Due to its texture, almond meal is not a substitute for blanched almond flour. Bob's Red Mill makes an excellent almond meal, and you can find a good one at Trader Joe's as well.

Coconut Flour

Coconut flour is naturally gluten-free, low in carbs, and high in fiber, which makes it an excellent choice for keto baking. It's made by dehydrating and then finely grinding the coconut meat into powder. However, it is a little trickier to work with because it is a very thirsty flour and therefore requires more eggs, liquids, or both. Recipes that use coconut flour usually use a smaller amount of it, since it is not a one-to-one substitute for nut flours. I use only coconut flour in my pancake recipes to get the fluffiest results.

Hazelnut Flour

Hazelnut flour (sometimes called hazelnut meal) is made from whole hazelnuts and is considered a meal rather than a flour, since the skin is left intact. It has a rich, sweet, nutty flavor and a denser texture than almond flour. This grain-free flour substitute is high in unsaturated fat and a good source of fiber and protein. My Hazelnut-Chocolate Snack Cakes (page 106) use hazelnut flour exclusively for a flavor-packed treat. You can find hazelnut flour at many health food stores and online retailers; my favorite is from Hazelnut Hill.

Sunflower Seed Flour

Sunflower seed flour is a byproduct of grinding sunflower seeds into a powder. Though sunflower seed flour is nut-free, it actually has a slightly nutty and sweet flavor and works as a one-to-one substitute for almond flour, which makes it an excellent candidate for nut-free keto baking. Sunflower seed flour can be found online from Thrive Market, Amazon, and other online retailers. You can also make sunflower seed flour by grinding sunflower seeds in a clean, dry coffee grinder, which can be more economical than buying it ready-made.

NUT-FREE KETO

If you need an allergen-free flour substitute, you have a few options. You can substitute nut flours, such as almond and hazelnut, one-to-one for either sesame seed or sunflower seed flour. However, it's crucial to source any nut-free flour substitute from a facility that does not also process nuts to prevent cross-contamination.

Coconut flour can also be an option if you have been cleared by your doctor to use it. However, coconut flour is much more absorbent than nut and seed flours, so it's not possible to substitute coconut flour for other flours at a one-to-one ratio. To substitute with coconut flour, you'll need to reduce the amount to a quarter of what the recipe calls for and add another egg to help with moisture and structure. One of my favorite recipes that I've developed using coconut flour is Double Chocolate Peppermint Cookies (page 97). They are rich in flavor and can be made quickly.

Flax meal is made from ground flaxseed, and it can be used in keto baking as a flour substitute or as an egg replacement. I prefer to use golden flax meal, as I find it less gummy than regular flax meal. Golden flax meal has an earthy, nutty flavor and gives recipes like my Flax Meal Tortillas (page 82) a nice flexible texture. Flax meal is easily found at most grocery stores now, and while golden flax is less common, it can still be found at most natural food stores and online retailers. My favorite brands to use are Bob's Red Mill and Whole Foods 365 Everyday Value organic.

SWEETENERS

You will notice that all the recipes use an erythritol blend as a sweetener. I favor erythritol in keto recipes because it does not get metabolized by the body and therefore has no effect on blood sugar levels. It's why it's not counted in the net carbohydrates in the recipes.

There are several erythritol blends on the market. In my recipes, I prefer to use Lakanto Monkfruit Sweetener, an erythritol–monk fruit blend, but if you prefer an erythritol-oligosaccharides blend, like Swerve, you can use the two interchangeably. Both brands have granulated, powdered, and brown sugar formulations.

BAKING CHOCOLATE AND UNSWEETENED COCOA POWDER

I love using baking chocolate and unsweetened cocoa powder in my keto dessert recipes. They both add rich chocolate flavor without adding sugar. Baking chocolate is naturally sugar-free and can be shaved finely or melted and folded into a batter. Natural unsweetened cocoa powder has a strong, bitter chocolate flavor, and the acid in the chocolate can act as a rising agent when it's used in recipes that call for baking soda.

EXTRACTS

Extracts can intensify or add a flavor punch without affecting macros very much, which is why I love to use them in my keto baked goods. A favorite in all baking, vanilla extract enhances all the flavors in a sweet recipe, much as salt does for savory dishes. When vanilla is left out of cookies, brownies, and other baked goods, I find they tend to taste flat and bland.

Lemon extract boosts the lemony flavor of recipes, especially when used with freshly grated lemon zest. Hazelnut extract is another great one to have on hand to enhance the nutty flavor of baked goods or to add the flavor without adding actual nuts (though I recommend double-checking the specific brand you're using to make sure it is indeed nut-free if needed). And then there are other more specialty extracts and flavorings you can buy from brands like One on One Flavors (OOOFlavors.com). It's easy to go wild on their site, but if you can only purchase one, I highly recommend their corn bread flavoring—it's key for making keto corn bread.

LEAVENING AGENTS

Leavening agents are what make dough rise so that your keto breads will be light and airy.

Yeast

Baker's yeast is used commonly in bread and other baked goods. It's a leavening agent that causes the dough to rise and become lighter via the fermentation process. In keto baking, yeast is used more for flavor; since we're using flours that have no gluten, the dough won't rise as much or be as stretchy. I recommend using instant dry yeast when keto baking, since it rises faster.

Inulin

Inulin, a prebiotic fiber found in starchy vegetables, can be used instead of regular sugar when proofing yeast. When proofing yeast with sugar, the sugar gets completely used up by the yeast in the proofing process and thus does not affect your carb count. However, many people still prefer not to use any sugar at all—partly because having regular sugar at home can be too tempting. Inulin can be used as a substitute for sugar in any keto recipe that uses yeast, such as my Cinnamon Rolls with Cream Cheese Icing (page 103) or Chorizo Bagels (page 50).

Baking Soda

Baking soda reacts with acidic ingredients, such as citrus juices and vinegar, to create carbon dioxide, which causes baked goods to rise. Be careful not to add more than a recipe calls for, though, because you'll get a soapy, metallic flavor.

Baking Powder

Baking powder is a mixture of baking soda and cream of tartar, an acid, which is why it doesn't require an acid to rise. Using fresh baking powder is crucial. Make sure to check the expiration date, and if you live in a humid environment, replace it sooner, since both baking powder and baking soda absorb a lot of moisture. I recommend using only gluten-free baking powder, such as Hain Featherweight.

SALT

Salt has several functions in baked goods. First of all, salt enhances the flavor in both savory and sweet dishes. Salt also plays a role in the texture of bread. Baked products without salt will taste flat, which is why it is used in keto baking, too.

In these recipes, I have specified sea salt (I prefer Himalayan) in a fine texture because regular table salt is heavily processed and eliminates many minerals that are beneficial in the ketogenic diet. However, you can use regular table salt in the recipes with the same baking results.

BINDERS

In the absence of gluten, binders are needed to hold keto baked goods together and give them a lighter texture.

Xanthan Gum

Xanthan gum is an excellent binder and helps to stabilize keto breads, much the way gluten does for traditional breads. Xanthan gum makes the dough sticky and traps the bubbles created by the leavening, which allows the dough to rise. This means your keto breads won't be a crumbly mess. It also makes for an excellent substitute for cornstarch, which is great for making keto cookies and brownies chewy. Though it may seem pricey, a little goes a long way. Usually, all you need is ½ teaspoon or less for xanthan gum to work its magic in a recipe. You can find xanthan gum in the baking section of most larger grocery stores or in the gluten-free baking section, if your store has one.

Eggs

Eggs are used in keto baking to help bind the ingredients and to help the dough rise. I recommend using pasture-raised and organic USDA grade AA or A large eggs. For the best results, use fresh eggs, and bring them to room temperature before using them. You can quickly do so by placing uncracked eggs in a bowl of hot water for 5 minutes.

Psyllium Husk Powder

The husk of the seed of the psyllium plant, an annual herb, contains a type of soluble fiber that absorbs liquid and produces a thick gel. It's prized in keto baking because the gel provides structure and volume in the absence of gluten. Some brands can cause baked products to have a harmless purple hue. I recommend using the NOW Foods brand found in natural food stores and from online retailers.

COCONUT OIL

Coconut oil is perfect for replacing traditional oils in keto baking. I use refined coconut oil in my baked goods because it can withstand higher temperatures and has a neutral taste. It's easy to work with; just make sure to check whether the recipe calls for it in its solid or liquid state. You can also replace butter with coconut oil to make your keto baked goods dairy-free.

DAIRY

Dairy products do contain some carbs, but the ones we use in baking are higher in fats and lower in sugar.

Butter

Butter is great for adding moisture and flavor to any kind of baked good, keto included. I usually recommend unsalted butter when baking because salted butter contains not only an unpredictable amount of salt but also more water. This could interact differently with your recipe and not allow for as much stability as unsalted butter. If you can, use butter from grass-fed cows because it contains omega-3 fatty acids, which are good for brain function and so much more.

Heavy Whipping Cream

Heavy cream makes for a great substitute for regular milk because it is much lower in carbs. Regular milk contains 12 grams of carbohydrates in just one cup, and heavy whipping cream has 7 grams. While that may not seem like a large difference, every little bit helps if you're trying to stay under 20 grams of carbs a day.

Cream Cheese

When it comes to keto baking, cream cheese is a game-changer. It's great for binding batters and giving stability. Your cream cheese should always be full-fat and at room temperature when baking unless the recipe says otherwise. You should also only use the cream cheese that comes in a block, not the whipped kind.

THE KETO BAKER'S EQUIPMENT

When it comes to keto baking, there isn't a lot of additional fancy equipment needed to achieve the perfect keto baked goods to keep you on track to a healthier you. You'll be happy to know that you can start making keto treats with what you already have on hand, except for maybe a few new items.

ESSENTIAL TOOLS

These are the essentials that you'll need to bake the delicious treats in this book. You probably already have most of them in your kitchen.

Mixing Bowls

The recipe you are making will determine the size as well as the material. They come in glass, ceramic, metal, and plastic, and each serves a specific purpose. Factors to consider when choosing which bowl to use include whether it is safe to put in the microwave, dishwasher, or freezer, as well as the capacity.

Measuring Cups and Spoons

Accurate measuring is vital in baking and can make or break your end result. Measuring cups for liquids are clear, typically glass or plastic, with graduated measurements. For dry ingredients, they come in sets with a cup for each measurement, usually 1 cup, ½ cup, ⅓ cup, and ¼ cup. I recommend a glass 2-cup measuring cup with a spout for liquids and stainless steel measuring cups for dry ingredients.

Measuring spoons come in a wide array of materials and sizes. It's best to have two sets, so you can measure dry and wet ingredients without stopping to clean and dry the spoons.

Stainless Steel Flour Sifter

Most of my nut flour recipes call for sifting to help break up any clumping and remove any larger pieces of nuts and skin left behind. Choose a sifter with a 3-cup capacity.

Cast Iron Skillet

My 9-inch cast iron skillet just might be the most beloved item in my kitchen. It's great for creating a perfect crust on corn bread or scones. That's because it's fabulous at retaining heat, which means it cooks more evenly and crisps to perfection. Be sure to buy a cast iron skillet that is preseasoned, and avoid rusting by never storing it wet.

Nonstick Muffin Pan

You will always be reaching for your 12-cup nonstick muffin pan when you're keto baking. It's perfect for portion control and makes meal planning a breeze. What's great about nonstick is that you don't always need to use paper liners, as long as you make sure to butter or grease the cups well.

Loaf Pan

A 9-by-5-inch loaf pan is essential for making keto breads, both savory and sweet. I am partial to metal loaf pans, since I have found that using glass for keto breads causes them to be soggy. I really like the Nordic Ware 1-pound loaf pan for my quick breads because it's a great nonstick choice.

Baking Sheets

Every keto baker needs a few good baking sheets. I like to use a 12-by-17-inch sheet pan, but what works for you will depend on the size of your oven. Cookie sheets are not rimmed all around, so they're great for cookies but impractical for many other items. Baking sheets are rimmed on all four sides, so they are also perfect for making keto flatbreads and free-form pizzas.

Square Baking Pan

An 8-by-8-inch square baking pan is the perfect size for making keto brownies and lots of other treats. You can get 16 perfect-size portions out of the 8-by-8 pan, and it's what I use most often when formulating my recipes—especially cookie bars.

Electric Hand Mixer

An electric hand mixer will make blending ingredients in keto baking much easier for more consistent results, especially when mixing heavier ingredients like cream cheese. Their small size makes them a light and portable choice compared to a stand mixer. They are also more economical. This book's recipes use an electric mixer, but you can use a stand mixer instead for any recipe with the same results.

Coffee Grinder

Although you can buy flax already milled, it is still not finely ground. That's why, in this book, I recommend that you grind the meal further in a coffee grinder. In larger quantities, flax meal that is not finely ground can make the recipe gummy.

The fastest, easiest, and most effective way to grind flax meal is in an electric coffee grinder (although you can use a spice grinder or even a mortar and pestle). You need a separate coffee grinder for this—not one you also use for coffee because it will have coffee oils on it, which will flavor the flax meal. You can also use this spare coffee grinder to grind whole spices.

IN THE UTILITY DRAWER

You probably already have a rubber spatula, a pancake turner, some wooden spoons, and a good chef's knife. A whisk is necessary to blend ingredients smoothly and add air to a mixture. A basic balloon whisk is really all you will need for the recipes here. I recommend using a stainless steel whisk, as they are faster and better at breaking up lumps than their silicone counterparts. You will also need parchment paper to line your pans and prevent sticking.

SPECIALTY ITEMS

Here are a few more items you can consider adding to your keto baking arsenal. They're not totally necessary but will make keto baking a little faster and smoother.

Cookie Scoops

Although cookie scoops are not essential, they can be useful to ensure uniform sizes and portions. A small scoop holds a little less than 1 ounce of dough and results in a baked cookie that is about 2 inches in diameter. A medium scoop holds about 1.25 ounces of dough and yields a 3-inch cookie. A large scoop can hold 2.25 ounces of dough and produces a 4-inch cookie. In this book, when I say "cookie scoop," I mean a small 1-ounce scoop.

Silicone Baking Mat

A silicone baking mat is meant to line a baking sheet to prevent sticking and burning. Although parchment paper and nonstick baking sprays serve this same purpose, sprays can be difficult to clean off your baking sheets, and parchment paper can be cumbersome and wasteful. Silicone baking mats are safe, easy to clean, and reusable.

Stand Mixer

Stand mixers make getting those nut flour–based batters nice and smooth. They also do a great job of blending my cream cheese–heavy recipes, which can be quite a task. My favorite is the KitchenAid Artisan stand mixer.

High-Powered Blender

A high-powered blender isn't just for smoothies. Having a high-powered blender makes creating a smooth pancake and waffle batter faster and easier—and it's easier to clean than a mixing bowl and electric mixer. I recommend the Vitamix Explorian blender for its multiple functions and high-speed options.

Waffle Iron

Of course, you need an electric waffle iron for all of the waffle recipes in this book. There are a variety of types and makers at various price points. I recommend a non-stick waffle maker, since the ingredients in keto waffles tend to stick more often than the ones in traditional recipes. You can use a classic or a Belgian waffle iron in all my recipes; just be sure to follow the manufacturer's instructions for cooking, as they tend to vary. And if you don't want to invest in a waffle iron, just use the waffle batter to make pancakes.

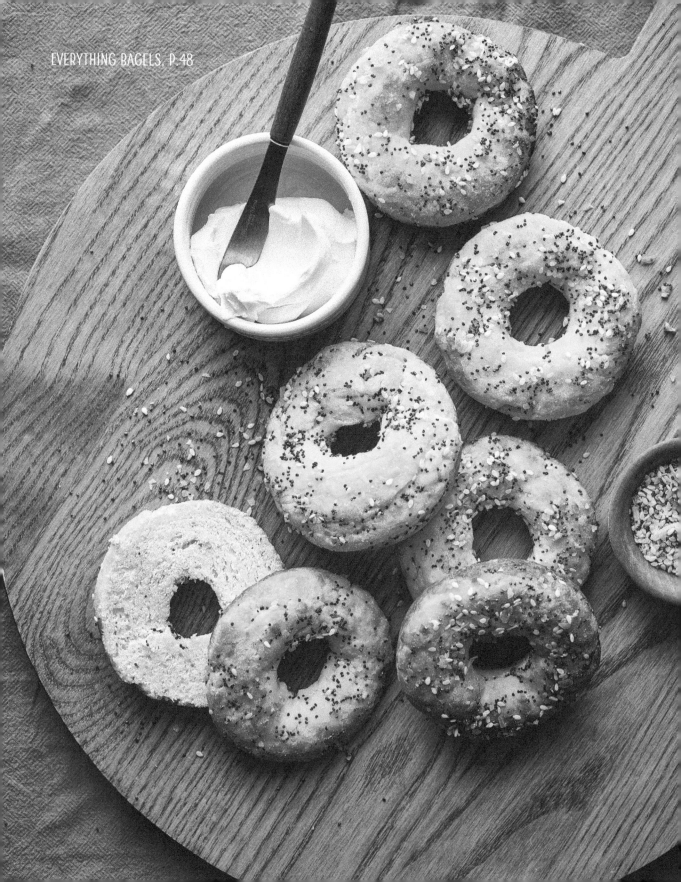

EVERYTHING BAGELS, P. 48

CHAPTER 3

ﮩﮩ

PANCAKES, WAFFLES, AND BREAKFAST BREADS

CHOCOLATE, CHOCOLATE CHIP PANCAKES

MAKES 10 PANCAKES / PREP TIME: 10 MINUTES / COOK TIME: 20 MINUTES
EQUIPMENT: 1 MIXING BOWL, HIGH-POWERED BLENDER OR ELECTRIC MIXER, NONSTICK SKILLET

Chocolate for breakfast? Why not? Some mornings require a little extra motivation, and chocolate chip pancakes are sure to get you going. The fact that these rich pancakes happen to be low enough in carbs to fit your daily macros, well, that's pure happiness. While I prefer to use a high-powered blender to mix all of my pancake and waffle batters, you can also use an electric mixer. Just be sure your cream cheese and eggs are fully combined before adding the dry ingredients to avoid lumps in your batter.

7 large eggs, at room temperature
8 ounces (about 1 cup) cream cheese, at room temperature
½ cup heavy whipping cream
1 teaspoon pure vanilla extract
½ cup granulated erythritol–monk fruit blend

½ cup coconut flour
¼ cup unsweetened cocoa powder
2 teaspoons baking powder
¼ teaspoon sea salt
2 to 3 tablespoons butter, divided
¼ cup sugar-free chocolate chips

1. Using a high-powered blender (or an electric mixer and a large mixing bowl), blend the eggs, cream cheese, heavy whipping cream, and vanilla until fully combined. Add the erythritol–monk fruit blend, coconut flour, cocoa powder, baking powder, and salt. Blend the pancake batter, being sure to stop to scrape down the sides of the blender or mixing bowl with a spatula a couple of times to ensure that the ingredients are well incorporated.

2. In a nonstick skillet over medium heat, melt 1 teaspoon of butter. Using a ladle, add about 3 tablespoons of batter to the hot skillet, and sprinkle a few chocolate chips over the top of the pancakes. Cook for about 2 minutes, or until bubbles start to form. Flip, and cook for another 1½ to 2 minutes or until fully cooked. Repeat with the rest of the batter, adding butter before each new ladle of batter.

3. Store any leftovers in the refrigerator for up to 5 days, or freeze for up to 3 weeks.

Keep in Mind: Keto pancake batter should be about the same consistency as traditional pancake batter. For all the pancake recipes in this chapter, if the batter is too thick, add more heavy whipping cream a tablespoon at a time until it is the right consistency.

Per serving: Calories: 249; Total Fat: 21g; Total Carbohydrates: 11g; Net Carbs: 7g; Fiber: 4g; Protein: 8g; Erythritol: 10g
Macros: Fat: 76%; Protein: 13%; Carbs: 11%

BLUEBERRY PANCAKES WITH BLUEBERRY SYRUP

MAKES 10 PANCAKES / PREP TIME: 10 MINUTES / COOK TIME: 20 MINUTES
EQUIPMENT: 1 MIXING BOWL, HIGH-POWERED BLENDER OR ELECTRIC MIXER, NONSTICK SKILLET, SAUCEPAN

I struggled with the idea that, on a keto diet, the fruit choices are limited. Thankfully, berries are on the safe list. It's best to stick to small servings and enjoy them in season. These blueberry pancakes are bursting with antioxidant-rich blueberries and are sure to satisfy any fruit cravings. And since you whip up these fluffy pancakes in a blender, they are also a breeze to make.

FOR THE BLUEBERRY SYRUP
2 tablespoons unsalted butter
¼ cup blueberries, fresh or frozen
½ cup sugar-free maple syrup

FOR THE PANCAKES
7 large eggs, at room temperature
8 ounces (about 1 cup) cream cheese, at room temperature
¼ cup heavy whipping cream
1 teaspoon pure vanilla extract
½ cup coconut flour
½ cup granulated erythritol–monk fruit blend
2 teaspoons baking powder
¼ teaspoon sea salt
2 to 3 tablespoons unsalted butter, divided
½ cup blueberries, fresh or frozen

TO MAKE THE BLUEBERRY SYRUP

1. Melt the butter on medium-low heat in a small saucepan. Add the blueberries, and stir until the berries pop and are incorporated into the butter.

2. Add the maple syrup, and allow the mixture to heat through but not boil for about 2 minutes. Set aside.

TO MAKE THE PANCAKES

1. Using a high-powered blender (or an electric mixer and a large mixing bowl), blend the eggs, cream cheese, heavy whipping cream, and vanilla until fully combined. Add the coconut flour, erythritol–monk fruit blend, baking powder, and salt. Blend or mix the pancake batter until it is well incorporated, being sure to stop to scrape down the sides of the blender or bowl with a rubber spatula a couple of times.

2. In a nonstick skillet over medium heat, melt 1 teaspoon of butter. Using a ladle, add about 3 tablespoons of batter to the hot skillet, and sprinkle a couple of blueberries over the top of the pancakes. Cook for about 2 minutes, or until bubbles start to form. Flip, and cook for another 1½ to 2 minutes, or until fully cooked. Repeat the process with the rest of the batter, adding more butter to the pan each time.

3. Serve topped with warm syrup.

4. Store any leftovers in the refrigerator for up to 5 days, or freeze for up to 3 weeks.

Ingredient Tip: If you're using frozen blueberries, let them defrost before adding them to pancakes.

Per serving: Calories: 224; Total Fat: 19g; Total Carbohydrates: 8g; Net Carbs: 5g; Fiber: 3g; Protein: 7g; Erythritol: 10g
Macros: Fat: 76%; Protein: 13%; Carbs: 11%

PUMPKIN PANCAKES WITH MAPLE CREAM CHEESE FROSTING

MAKES 10 PANCAKES / PREP TIME: 10 MINUTES / COOK TIME: 20 MINUTES
EQUIPMENT: 2 MIXING BOWLS, HIGH-POWERED BLENDER, ELECTRIC MIXER, NONSTICK SKILLET

I love making pumpkin pancakes full of fall spices on chilly weekend mornings. The smell of pumpkin is intoxicating. And when these pancakes are heaped with a dollop of maple cream cheese frosting, they become a decadent treat. It's one you will want to enjoy all autumn long.

FOR THE MAPLE CREAM CHEESE FROSTING

4 ounces (about ½ cup) cream cheese, at room temperature
½ cup confectioners' erythritol–monk fruit blend
¼ cup sugar-free maple syrup
2 tablespoons heavy whipping cream
½ teaspoon pure vanilla extract
¼ teaspoon ground cinnamon
⅛ teaspoon sea salt

FOR THE PANCAKES

7 large eggs, at room temperature
8 ounces (about 1 cup) cream cheese, at room temperature
½ cup canned pumpkin purée
¼ cup heavy whipping cream
1 teaspoon pure vanilla extract
½ cup coconut flour
½ cup granulated erythritol–monk fruit blend
2 teaspoons baking powder
2 teaspoons ground cinnamon
½ teaspoon ground ginger
¼ teaspoon ground nutmeg
Pinch ground cloves
¼ teaspoon sea salt
2 to 3 tablespoons butter, divided

TO MAKE THE MAPLE CREAM CHEESE FROSTING

Using an electric mixer and medium mixing bowl, combine the cream cheese, erythritol–monk fruit blend, maple syrup, heavy whipping cream, vanilla, cinnamon, and salt, and blend until they have a creamy consistency and are fully combined. Set aside.

TO MAKE THE PANCAKES

1. Using a high-powered blender (or an electric mixer and a large mixing bowl), blend the eggs, cream cheese, pumpkin purée, heavy whipping cream, and vanilla, and process until fully combined. Add the coconut flour, erythritol–monk fruit blend, baking powder, cinnamon, ginger, nutmeg, cloves, and salt. Mix the pancake batter, being sure to stop to scrape down the sides of the blender or bowl a couple of times with a rubber spatula to ensure that the batter is well incorporated.

2. In a nonstick skillet over medium heat, melt 1 teaspoon of butter. Using a ladle, add about 3 tablespoons of batter to the hot skillet. Cook for about 2 minutes, or until bubbles start to form. Flip, and cook for another 1½ to 2 minutes, or until fully cooked. Repeat the process with the rest of the batter, adding butter to the pan each time.

3. Serve spread with the frosting.

4. Store any leftovers in the refrigerator for up to 5 days, or freeze for up to 3 weeks.

Ingredient Tip: Be sure to buy pure plain pumpkin purée, not pumpkin pie filling, which contains sugar and spices.

Per serving: Calories: 252; Total Fat: 21g; Total Carbohydrates: 9g; Net Carbs: 6g; Fiber: 3g; Protein: 8g; Erythritol: 17g
Macros: Fat: 75%; Protein: 13%; Carbs: 12%

VERY BERRY WAFFLES

MAKES 4 WAFFLES / PREP TIME: 10 MINUTES / COOK TIME: 25 TO 35 MINUTES
EQUIPMENT: 2 MIXING BOWLS, ELECTRIC MIXER, WAFFLE IRON

These delicious waffles start with a basic fail-proof waffle recipe and then are topped with a triple dose of berries in the form of a quick sauce. The fact that this recipe comes together rather easily means you can make them part of your regular keto meal rotation. If you don't have a waffle iron, use this batter to make delicious pancakes.

FOR THE MIXED BERRY TOPPING
½ cup water
¼ cup blueberries, fresh or frozen
¼ cup raspberries, fresh or frozen
¼ cup chopped strawberries
¼ cup granulated erythritol–monk fruit blend

FOR THE WAFFLES
1 cup finely milled almond flour, measured and sifted
¼ cup coconut flour
¼ cup granulated erythritol–monk fruit blend
1 tablespoon psyllium husk powder
2 teaspoons baking powder
¼ teaspoon sea salt
8 ounces (about 1 cup) cream cheese, at room temperature
1 teaspoon pure vanilla extract
5 large eggs, at room temperature
½ to ¾ cup water
2 tablespoons unsalted butter, melted

TO MAKE THE MIXED BERRY TOPPING
In a small saucepan over medium-low heat, gently simmer the water, blueberries, raspberries, strawberries, and erythritol–monk fruit blend for 7 to 10 minutes, or until the sauce reduces and thickens.

TO MAKE THE WAFFLES

1. Preheat the waffle iron.

2. In a large bowl, whisk together the almond flour, coconut flour, erythritol–monk fruit blend, psyllium husk powder, baking powder, and salt. Set aside.

3. In a medium bowl, combine the cream cheese and vanilla. Add the eggs one at a time, mixing after each egg is added.

4. Add the egg mixture to the dry ingredients, and combine using a rubber spatula. Add ½ cup water, and stir to combine. Add up to another ¼ cup water as needed—the batter thickens as it sits.

5. Grease a waffle iron well with the melted butter. Add spoonfuls of batter evenly, being sure not to overfill the waffle iron. Close the waffle iron, and cook according to the manufacturer's instructions. Serve the waffles topped with mixed berry topping.

6. Store any leftovers in an airtight container in the refrigerator for up to 5 days, or freeze for up to 3 weeks. Reheat in a toaster or toaster oven set to medium heat.

Variation Tip: For a faster and easier berry sauce, you can combine ¼ cup sugar-free strawberry jelly with 2 tablespoons butter, and heat for 30-second increments in the microwave or on the stovetop using a saucepan over medium heat for 5 to 7 minutes, or until it melts and thickens into a sauce.

Per serving: Calories: 551; Total Fat: 46g; Total Carbohydrates: 20g; Net Carbs: 11g; Fiber: 9g; Protein: 19g; Erythritol: 24g
Macros: Fat: 75%; Protein: 14%; Carbs: 11%

HAM AND SWISS WAFFLES

MAKES 4 WAFFLES / PREP TIME: 10 MINUTES / COOK TIME: 25 TO 35 MINUTES
EQUIPMENT: 2 MIXING BOWLS, ELECTRIC MIXER, WAFFLE IRON

Savory waffles? Don't knock it till you try it! These ham and Swiss cheese waffles are delicious with some sugar-free syrup for that perfect sweet-salty combo. They make for a great sandwich alternative, too. As an added bonus, these waffles freeze beautifully, so you can make a big batch and pop your waffles straight from your freezer into your toaster on busy weekdays.

1 cup finely milled almond flour, measured and sifted
¼ cup coconut flour
2 tablespoons granulated erythritol–monk fruit blend
1 tablespoon psyllium husk powder
2 teaspoons baking powder
½ teaspoon sea salt
¼ teaspoon black pepper

8 ounces (about 1 cup) cream cheese, at room temperature
1 teaspoon pure vanilla extract
5 large eggs, at room temperature
¼ cup finely chopped ham
¼ cup finely chopped Swiss cheese
½ to ¾ cup water
2 tablespoons unsalted butter, melted

1. Preheat the waffle iron.

2. In a large bowl, whisk together the almond flour, coconut flour, erythritol–monk fruit blend, psyllium husk powder, baking powder, salt, and pepper, and set aside.

3. In a medium bowl, using an electric mixer, combine the cream cheese and vanilla. Add the eggs one at a time, mixing after each egg is added.

4. Add the egg mixture to the dry ingredients using a rubber spatula. Fold in the ham and Swiss cheese. Add ½ cup water, and stir to combine. Add up to another ¼ cup water as needed—the batter thickens as it sits.

5. Grease a waffle iron well with the melted butter. Add spoonfuls of batter evenly, being sure not to overfill the waffle iron. Close the waffle iron, and cook according to the manufacturer's instructions.

6. Store any leftovers in an airtight container in the refrigerator for up to 5 days, or freeze for up to 3 weeks. Reheat in the toaster or toaster oven set to medium heat.

Variation Tip: For a different flavor profile, substitute Cheddar cheese and cooked bacon for the ham and Swiss. And if you don't have a waffle iron, just use this batter to make pancakes.

Per serving: Calories: 583; Total Fat: 49g; Total Carbohydrates: 17g; Net Carbs: 9g; Fiber: 8g; Protein: 23g; Erythritol: 6g
Macros: Fat: 76%; Protein: 16%; Carbs: 8%

DAIRY-FREE CHURRO MUFFINS

MAKES 12 MUFFINS / PREP TIME: 5 TO 10 MINUTES / COOK TIME: 20 TO 25 MINUTES, PLUS 10 MINUTES TO COOL
EQUIPMENT: 3 MIXING BOWLS, ELECTRIC MIXER, 12-CUP MUFFIN PAN

These muffins are a sweet cinnamon Mexican dessert in a baked (not fried, as churros usually are) low-carb treat. These little muffins are also dairy-free, giving you a delicious and easy option that even the dairy-sensitive can enjoy. These make for a tasty morning breakfast treat, but that's not to say you can't have them any time of day as a great snack.

FOR THE CHURRO TOPPING
⅓ cup granulated erythritol–monk fruit blend
2 teaspoons ground cinnamon

FOR THE MUFFINS
¾ cup granulated erythritol–monk fruit blend
½ cup coconut oil, solid
2 large eggs, at room temperature
¼ cup coconut or almond milk
½ teaspoon pure vanilla extract
1½ cups finely milled almond flour, measured and sifted
1¼ teaspoons baking powder
1 teaspoon ground cinnamon
¼ teaspoon ground nutmeg
¼ teaspoon sea salt

TO MAKE THE CHURRO TOPPING
In a small bowl, combine the granulated erythritol–monk fruit blend and cinnamon. Set aside.

TO MAKE THE MUFFINS
1. Preheat the oven to 350°F. Line a 12-cup muffin pan with cupcake liners, or grease each opening.

2. In a large bowl, using an electric mixer, cream the erythritol–monk fruit blend and coconut oil until light and fluffy. Beat in the eggs one at a time. Add the coconut milk and vanilla, and combine well.

3. In a medium bowl, combine the almond flour, baking powder, cinnamon, nutmeg, and salt. Add the dry ingredients to the wet ingredients, and mix well.

4. Scoop or pour the batter into the muffin cups until they are mostly full. Sprinkle the churro topping evenly on top of the muffins before baking.

5. Bake for 20 to 25 minutes, or until a toothpick inserted into the center comes out clean. Allow the muffins to cool in the pan for 10 minutes and then transfer to a wire rack to cool thoroughly.

6. Store any leftovers in an airtight container in the refrigerator for up to 5 days, or freeze for up to 3 weeks.

Variation Tip: For a Mexican hot chocolate flavor profile, add 1 teaspoon unsweetened cocoa powder to the churro topping.

Per serving: Calories: 176; Total Fat: 17g; Total Carbohydrates: 4g; Net Carbs: 2g; Fiber: 2g; Protein: 4g; Erythritol: 17g
Macros: Fat: 87%; Protein: 9%; Carbs: 4%

GLAZED DAIRY-FREE CARROT CAKE MUFFINS

MAKES 18 MUFFINS / PREP TIME: 10 MINUTES / COOK TIME: 20 TO 25 MINUTES, PLUS 15 MINUTES TO COOL
EQUIPMENT: 3 MIXING BOWLS, ELECTRIC MIXER, 2 (12-CUP) MUFFIN PANS

With the perfect balance of warm spices, these dairy-free carrot muffins are sure to satisfy your carrot cake cravings. Moist, tender, and full of flavor, this is a great portable breakfast option. And since they freeze well, you can make them on the weekend for busy weekdays.

FOR THE MUFFINS

1 cup coconut oil, melted and cooled
¾ cup brown or golden erythritol–monk fruit blend
5 large eggs, at room temperature
½ cup coconut milk
1 teaspoon pure vanilla extract
2 cups loosely packed grated carrots
2½ cups finely milled almond flour, measured and sifted
2 tablespoons ground cinnamon
2½ teaspoons baking powder
2 teaspoons ground ginger
½ teaspoon ground nutmeg
¼ teaspoon sea salt
¼ teaspoon ground cardamom
1 cup roughly chopped pecans
½ cup unsweetened coconut flakes

FOR THE VANILLA GLAZE

1 cup confectioners' erythritol–monk fruit blend
½ teaspoon pure vanilla extract
3 to 4 tablespoons coconut milk

TO MAKE THE MUFFINS

1. Preheat the oven to 365°F. Add 18 cupcake liners to 2 (12-cup) muffin pans (some cups will be empty), or grease 18 muffin openings.

2. In a large bowl, using a wooden spoon or electric mixer, cream the coconut oil and erythritol–monk fruit blend. Add the eggs one at a time, mixing well with each addition. Add the coconut milk and vanilla. Combine well. Add the carrots, and mix well. Set aside.

3. In a medium bowl, mix together the almond flour, cinnamon, baking powder, ginger, nutmeg, salt, and cardamom.

4. Add the dry ingredients to the wet ingredients, and mix until fully combined. Fold in the pecans and coconut flakes.

5. Scoop or pour the batter into the muffin cups until they are mostly full. Bake for 20 to 25 minutes, or until a toothpick inserted into the center comes out clean.

6. Allow the cupcakes to cool completely on a wire rack, about 15 minutes, before glazing.

TO MAKE THE VANILLA GLAZE AND FINISH THE MUFFINS

1. While the muffins are baking, combine the erythritol–monk fruit blend and vanilla in a small bowl. Add the coconut milk, starting with 3 tablespoons. Add another tablespoon if the glaze is too thick.

2. Once the muffins have completely cooled, drizzle the glaze on top. Don't add the glaze before the muffins are completely cooled or it will melt. If you are going to freeze them, leave off the glaze.

3. Store any leftovers in the refrigerator for up to 5 days, or freeze for up to 3 weeks.

Per serving: Calories: 304; Total Fat: 29g; Total Carbohydrates: 8g; Net Carbs: 4g; Fiber: 4g; Protein: 6g; Erythritol: 16g
Macros: Fat: 86%; Protein: 8%; Carbs: 6%

GLAZED CRANBERRY-ORANGE MUFFINS

MAKES 18 MUFFINS / PREP TIME: 10 MINUTES / COOK TIME: 20 TO 30 MINUTES, PLUS 15 MINUTES TO COOL
EQUIPMENT: 3 MIXING BOWLS, ELECTRIC MIXER, 2 (12-CUP)MUFFIN PANS

Bursting with cranberry and orange flavor, these moist muffins make for the perfect portable breakfast or afternoon snack. The zesty orange glaze drizzled over the top takes them to the next level. They will make a great addition to your keto breakfast rotation.

FOR THE MUFFINS
1¼ cups finely milled almond flour, measured and sifted
1½ teaspoons baking powder
¼ teaspoon sea salt
4 ounces (about ½ cup) cream cheese, at room temperature
4 tablespoons (½ stick) unsalted butter, at room temperature
¾ cup granulated erythritol–monk fruit blend
1 tablespoon grated orange zest
½ teaspoon liquid orange extract
4 large eggs, at room temperature
1 cup cranberries, fresh or frozen

FOR THE ORANGE GLAZE
½ cup confectioners' erythritol–monk fruit blend
1½ tablespoons freshly squeezed lemon juice
1 tablespoon heavy whipping cream
1 teaspoon freshly grated orange zest
½ teaspoon liquid orange extract

TO MAKE THE MUFFINS

1. Preheat the oven to 350°F. Add 18 cupcake liners to the 2 (12-cup) muffin pans (some cups will be empty), or grease 18 muffin openings.

2. In a medium bowl, whisk together the almond flour, baking powder, and salt.

3. In a large bowl, using an electric mixer, beat the cream cheese and butter on high speed until light and fluffy. Add the erythritol–monk fruit blend, orange zest, and orange extract, and whisk until combined. Add the eggs one at a time to the wet ingredients, mixing after each addition. Mix until they are well incorporated.

4. Add the dry ingredients to the wet batter, and blend until fully combined. Fold in the cranberries.

5. Scoop or pour the batter into the muffin cups until they are a little more than three-quarters full. (Depending on how deep your muffin pan is, you may have leftover batter that can fill some of the empty muffin cups.) Bake for 20 to 28 minutes, or until a toothpick inserted into the center comes out clean. Allow to cool completely on a wire rack for about 15 minutes before glazing.

TO MAKE THE ORANGE GLAZE AND FINISH THE MUFFINS

1. In a medium bowl, whisk together the erythritol–monk fruit blend, lemon juice, heavy whipping cream, orange zest, and orange extract until fully combined.

2. Once the muffins have completely cooled, drizzle the glaze on top. Don't add the glaze before the muffins are cool, or it will melt. If you are going to freeze them, leave off the glaze.

3. Store any leftovers in the refrigerator for up to 5 days, or freeze for up to 3 weeks.

Ingredient Tip: Use only an organic orange for the zest to avoid consuming pesticides. First, use a fruit and vegetable wash to clean the skin of the orange thoroughly. Next, using a box grater or a flat grater, scrape just the surface of the orange. Be careful not to get any of the bitter white pith.

Per serving: Calories: 111; Total Fat: 10g; Total Carbohydrates: 3g; Net Carbs: 2g; Fiber: 1g; Protein: 4g; Erythritol: 12g
Macros: Fat: 81%; Protein: 14%; Carbs: 5%

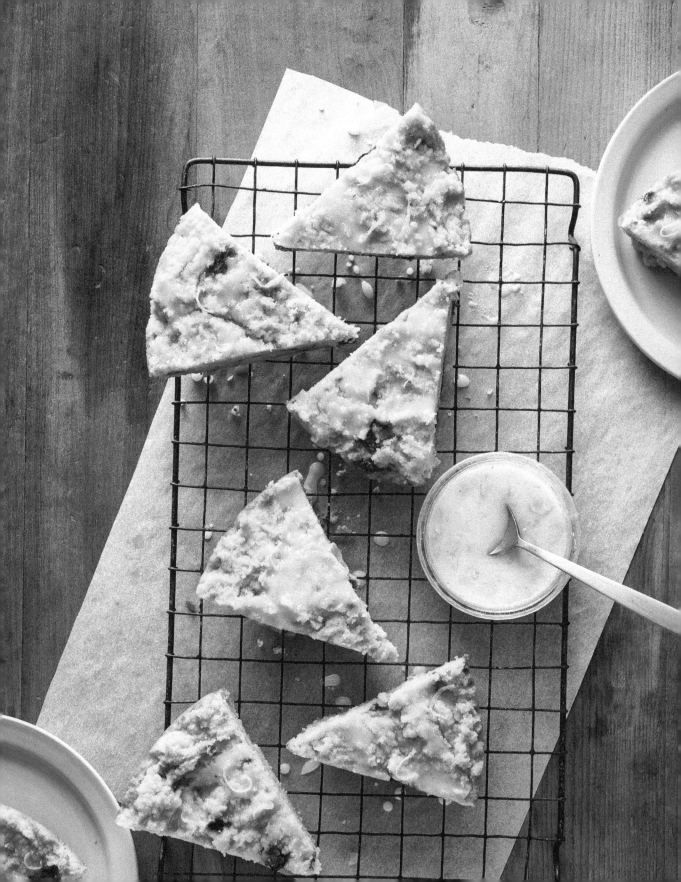

MIXED BERRY SCONES WITH LEMON ICING

MAKES 10 SCONES / PREP TIME: 10 MINUTES / COOK TIME: 25 TO 30 MINUTES, PLUS COOLING TIME
EQUIPMENT: 2 MIXING BOWLS, ELECTRIC MIXER, 9-INCH CAST IRON SKILLET

Mornings are sweeter with these mixed berry scones, whether you serve them during the week or on lazy weekends. These scones are bursting with antioxidant-rich berries and a lemony zing and are sure to satisfy the need for something delicious to accompany your coffee or tea. If you don't have a 9-inch cast iron skillet, a 9-inch round cake pan will also work.

FOR THE SCONES

4 tablespoons (½ stick) unsalted butter, melted and cooled, plus 1 tablespoon to grease the pan
½ cup granulated erythritol–monk fruit blend
½ teaspoon liquid lemon extract
3 large eggs, at room temperature
½ cup full-fat sour cream
1½ cups finely milled almond flour, measured and sifted
½ cup coconut flour
1½ teaspoons baking powder
¼ teaspoon sea salt
¼ cup blueberries, fresh or frozen
¼ cup raspberries, fresh or frozen
¼ cup chopped strawberries, fresh or frozen

FOR THE LEMON ICING

½ cup confectioners' erythritol–monk fruit blend
2 tablespoons freshly squeezed lemon juice
½ teaspoon liquid lemon extract
1 to 2 tablespoons heavy whipping cream
½ tablespoon grated lemon zest

TO MAKE THE SCONES

1. Preheat the oven to 375°F. Grease a 9-inch cast iron skillet with butter.

2. In a large bowl, using an electric mixer, combine the butter, erythritol–monk fruit blend, lemon extract, and eggs. Add the sour cream, and mix well. Add the almond flour, coconut flour, baking powder, and salt, and stir until fully combined. Fold the blueberries, raspberries, and strawberries into the batter.

Continued →

3. Spread the batter evenly in the skillet. Bake for 25 to 30 minutes, or until a tooth-pick inserted into the center comes out clean. Allow to cool completely in the skillet, then cut into wedges.

TO MAKE THE LEMON ICING AND FINISH THE SCONES

1. In a medium bowl, combine the erythritol–monk fruit blend, lemon juice, and lemon extract. Add the heavy whipping cream, starting with 1 tablespoon. Add another tablespoon if the icing is too thick.

2. Once the scones have fully cooled, drizzle with the icing, then sprinkle the lemon zest on top.

3. Store any leftovers in the refrigerator for up to 5 days, or freeze for up to 3 weeks.

Ingredient Tip: If you're using frozen berries, you do not need to defrost them before adding them to the batter.

Per serving: Calories: 232; Total Fat: 19g; Total Carbohydrates: 10g; Net Carbs: 5g; Fiber: 5g; Protein: 7g; Erythritol: 17g
Macros: Fat: 74%; Protein: 12%; Carbs: 14%

BACON CHEDDAR CHIVE SCONES

MAKES 10 SCONES / PREP TIME: 10 MINUTES / COOK TIME: 25 TO 30 MINUTES, PLUS COOLING TME
EQUIPMENT: 1 MIXING BOWL, ELECTRIC MIXER, 9-INCH CAST IRON SKILLET

If the words "bacon" and "Cheddar" didn't grab your attention, perhaps the fact that these scones are also light and fluffy will. Savory scones are just as delicious as their sweet counterparts, and in the case of these scones, they are also low in carbs and super easy to make.

4 tablespoons (¼ stick) unsalted butter, melted and cooled, plus 1 tablespoon to grease the pan

½ cup full-fat sour cream

3 large eggs, at room temperature

1½ cups finely milled almond flour, measured and sifted

½ cup coconut flour

1½ teaspoons baking powder

½ teaspoon sea salt

4 tablespoons shredded Cheddar cheese, divided

4 slices cooked bacon, crumbled, divided

2 tablespoons chopped chives

1. Preheat the oven to 375°F. Grease a 9-inch cast iron skillet with butter.

2. In a large bowl, using an electric mixer, combine the butter, sour cream, and eggs. Fold in the almond flour, coconut flour, baking powder, and salt with a rubber spatula until fully combined. Then fold in 2 tablespoons of Cheddar cheese and 2 slices of cooked crumbled bacon.

3. Spread the batter in the skillet. Sprinkle the remaining 2 tablespoons of Cheddar cheese, remaining 2 slices of bacon, and the chives on top.

4. Bake for 25 to 30 minutes, or until a toothpick inserted into the center comes out clean. Allow to cool completely in the skillet, then cut into wedges to serve.

5. Store any leftovers in the refrigerator for up to 5 days, or freeze for up to 3 weeks.

Keep in Mind: If you don't own the right size cast iron skillet, you can use a greased round 9-inch cake pan.

Per serving: Calories: 250; Total Fat: 21g; Total Carbohydrates: 9g; Net Carbs: 5g; Fiber: 4g; Protein: 9g; Erythritol: 0g

Macros: Fat: 76%; Protein: 14%; Carbs: 10%

CINNAMON FRENCH TOAST STICKS

MAKES 16 STICKS / PREP TIME: 15 MINUTES / COOK TIME: 35 TO 45 MINUTES, PLUS 15 TO 20 MINUTES TO COOL
EQUIPMENT: 2 MIXING BOWLS, COFFEE GRINDER, LARGE BAKING SHEET, LARGE SKILLET

Anytime I can have an excuse to eat with my fingers, I'm all in. Maybe it's a sensory thing, but it feels a little more indulgent when I'm enjoying food without utensils. These cinnamon toast sticks remind me of the donuts you find at the county fair, except that these are keto-friendly and therefore guilt-free.

3 tablespoons golden flax meal

1½ cups almond flour

5 tablespoons granulated erythritol–monk fruit blend, divided

1 tablespoon psyllium husk powder

2 teaspoons baking powder

¼ teaspoon sea salt

⅛ teaspoon xanthan gum

1 cup warm water

4 large eggs, at room temperature, divided

1 tablespoon coconut oil, melted

½ cup heavy whipping cream

1 teaspoon ground cinnamon

1 teaspoon pure vanilla extract

3 tablespoons butter, divided

Sugar-free maple syrup (optional)

1. Preheat the oven to 375°F. Line a large baking sheet with parchment paper or a silicone baking mat.

2. Grind the flax meal in a coffee grinder until it's a fine powder.

3. In a large bowl, combine the almond flour, flax meal powder, 3 tablespoons of erythritol–monk fruit blend, the psyllium husk powder, baking powder, salt, and xanthan gum. Add the warm water, 2 eggs, and the coconut oil, and combine well using a rubber spatula to make a dough.

4. Spread the dough onto the prepared baking sheet using a wet spatula.

5. Bake for 25 to 30 minutes, or until lightly browned. Allow to cool on a wire rack for 15 to 20 minutes before slicing.

6. Using a pizza cutter or sharp knife, cut the baked dough in half horizontally and then into 1½-inch strips vertically. You should have 2 rows of 6 sticks, for a total of 12 French toast sticks.

7. In a small bowl, prepare the egg wash by whisking the remaining 2 eggs, the heavy whipping cream, cinnamon, the remaining 2 tablespoons of erythritol–monk fruit blend, and the vanilla.

8. In a large skillet over medium heat, melt 1 tablespoon of butter. Dip 4 French toast sticks in the egg batter, and cook until lightly golden brown on both sides, or for 4 to 5 minutes total. Repeat with the remaining butter, French toast sticks, and batter. Serve immediately with sugar-free maple syrup (if using).

9. Store any leftovers in the refrigerator for up to 5 days, or freeze for up to 3 weeks. Reheat in a toaster oven.

Variation Tip: If you're not in the mood for a sweet dish, omit the egg batter, and just slice the baked bread into 4-by-4-inch squares perfect for grilled cheese and small sandwiches.

Per serving: Calories: 139; Total Fat: 13g; Total Carbohydrates: 4g; Net Carbs: 2g; Fiber: 2g; Protein: 4g; Erythritol: 4g
Macros: Fat: 84%; Protein: 12%; Carbs: 4%

EVERYTHING BAGELS

MAKES 8 BAGELS / PREP TIME: 20 MINUTES, PLUS RISING TIME / COOK TIME: 15 TO 20 MINUTES
EQUIPMENT: 2 MIXING BOWLS, LARGE BAKING SHEET

These delicious bagels have everything you love about traditional bagels, minus all the carbs. It uses a mozzarella dough, a favorite in the keto community, and gets an upgrade with the inclusion of yeast and a few other key ingredients. These everything bagels have both the flavor and texture of gluten bagels, but none of their sugar-spiking properties.

1 tablespoon yeast

1 teaspoon inulin fiber or sugar

3 tablespoons warm water

2 cups shredded part-skim mozzarella cheese

2 tablespoons cream cheese, at room temperature

¾ cup coconut flour

2 teaspoons baking powder

¼ teaspoon xanthan gum

2 large eggs, at room temperature

2 tablespoons unsalted butter, melted

1 tablespoon Trader Joe's Everything Bagel Topping or coarse sea salt

1. Line a large baking sheet with parchment paper or a silicone baking mat.

2. Proof the yeast: Put the yeast and inulin fiber in a small bowl (make sure the bowl is large enough to allow the yeast to expand). Add the warm water, and stir. Cover the bowl with a kitchen towel and leave to rest for 10 minutes. The yeast has properly proofed when it expands and bubbles.

3. Put the mozzarella cheese in a large microwave-safe bowl. Microwave in 30-second increments, making sure to stir each time, until fully melted. Add the cream cheese to the melted mozzarella, and mix until combined. Add the coconut flour, baking powder, and xanthan gum, and mix well using a rubber spatula. Add the eggs and the proofed yeast, and mix.

4. Once the dough comes together, with wet hands, lightly knead the dough. Divide the dough into 8 equal balls. On the prepared baking sheet, using wet hands, form the bagels and smooth any cracks on the surface or sides. Brush the tops and sides of bagels with the melted butter. Allow the bagels to rest and slightly rise in a warm, draft-free place for 30 to 45 minutes.

5. While the bagels are rising, preheat the oven to 375°F.

6. After rising, sprinkle the bagels with the everything bagel topping. Bake for 18 to 20 minutes, or until the bagels are golden brown.

7. Store any leftovers in the refrigerator for up to 7 days, or freeze for up to 3 weeks.

Ingredient Tip: If you don't have a Trader Joe's nearby, you can make your own everything bagel topping. Simply combine ¼ cup sesame seeds, ¼ cup poppy seeds, 3 tablespoons dried onion flakes, 3 tablespoons dried garlic flakes, and 2 tablespoons coarse salt. You can store this homemade everything bagel topping in an airtight container for up to 1 month.

Per serving: Calories: 191; Total Fat: 12g; Total Carbohydrates: 9g; Net Carbs: 4g; Fiber: 5g; Protein: 11g; Erythritol: 0g
Macros: Fat: 57%; Protein: 23%; Carbs: 20%

CHORIZO BAGELS

MAKES 8 BAGELS / PREP TIME: 20 MINUTES, PLUS RISING TIME / COOK TIME: 15 TO 20 MINUTES
EQUIPMENT: 2 MIXING BOWLS, LARGE BAKING SHEET

These tasty bagels start with my perfected mozzarella dough that includes yeast for both flavor and texture. The added bits of chorizo give them a delicious Spanish twist that will have you dancing in your kitchen. But seriously, these bagels are a must-try if you've been missing traditional bagels while doing keto.

1 tablespoon yeast

1 teaspoon inulin fiber or sugar

3 tablespoons warm water

2 cups shredded part-skim mozzarella cheese

2 tablespoons cream cheese, at room temperature

¾ cup coconut flour

2 teaspoons baking powder

¼ teaspoon xanthan gum

2 large eggs, at room temperature

¼ cup finely chopped fully cured Spanish chorizo, casing removed

2 tablespoons unsalted butter, melted

Coarse sea salt

1. Line a large baking sheet with parchment paper or a silicone baking mat.

2. Proof the yeast: Put the yeast and inulin fiber in a small bowl (make sure the bowl is large enough to allow the yeast to expand). Add the warm water and stir. Cover the bowl with a kitchen towel, and leave to rest for 10 minutes. The yeast has properly proofed when it expands and bubbles.

3. Put the mozzarella cheese in a large microwave-safe bowl. Microwave in 30-second increments, making sure to stir each time, until fully melted. Add the cream cheese to the melted mozzarella, and mix until combined.

4. Add the coconut flour, baking powder, and xanthan gum, and mix well using a rubber spatula. Add the eggs, chorizo, and proofed yeast, and combine well.

5. Once the dough comes together, with wet hands, lightly knead the dough. Divide the dough into 8 equal balls. On the prepared baking sheet, using wet hands, form the bagels, and smooth any cracks on the surface or sides. Brush the tops and sides of the bagels with the melted butter. Allow the bagels to rest and slightly rise in a warm, draft-free place for 30 to 45 minutes.

6. While the bagels are rising, preheat the oven to 375°F.

7. After rising, sprinkle the bagels with coarse sea salt. Bake for 18 to 20 minutes, or until the bagels are golden brown.

8. Store any leftovers in the refrigerator for up to 7 days, or freeze for up to 3 weeks.

Ingredient tip: Fully cured chorizo is dry-cured, meaning it is allowed to dry out for a period of time until it becomes harder in texture. It is eaten sliced, and there is no need to cook it. Can't find chorizo? Substitute 2 tablespoons cooked chopped bacon.

Per serving: Calories: 204; Total Fat: 13g; Total Carbohydrates: 10g; Net Carbs: 5g; Fiber: 5g; Protein: 13g; Erythritol: 0g
Macros: Fat: 57%; Protein: 25%; Carbs: 18%

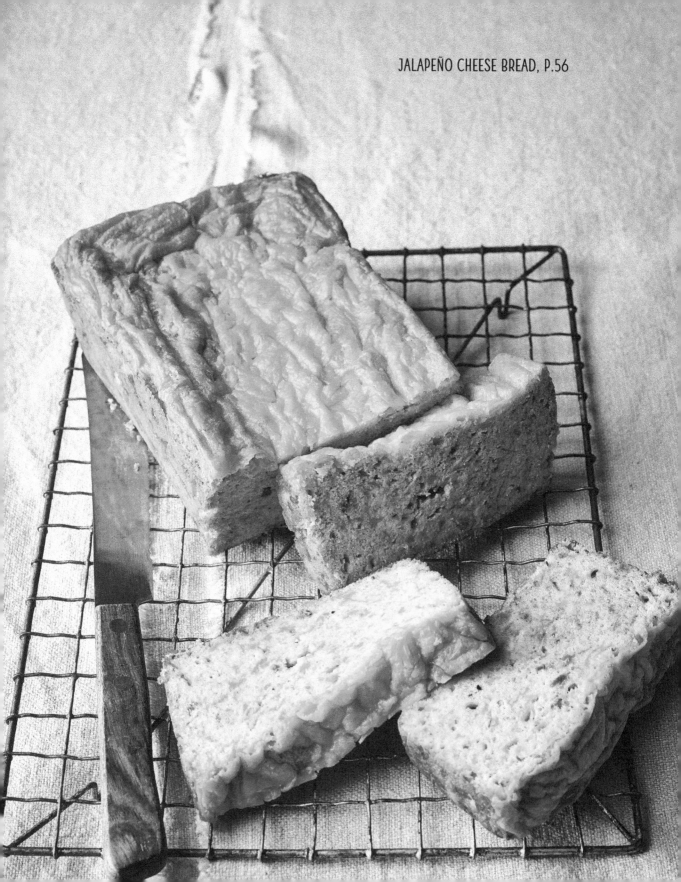

JALAPEÑO CHEESE BREAD, P.56

CHAPTER 4

~ﾑﾑﾑ~

SANDWICH BREADS, BISCUITS, AND BUNS

BASIC SANDWICH BREAD

MAKES 12 SLICES / PREP TIME: 10 MINUTES / COOK TIME: 30 TO 40 MINUTES, PLUS 30 TO 40 MINUTES TO COOL
EQUIPMENT: 2 MIXING BOWLS, ELECTRIC MIXER, 9-BY-5-INCH LOAF PAN

Every person following the keto diet needs an excellent basic sandwich bread. This recipe makes a light, fluffy option that is perfect for slicing, toasting, and of course, sandwiches. This bread freezes beautifully, so you can always have some on hand for when the cravings hit and you just need a sandwich.

1¼ cups finely milled almond flour, measured and sifted

1 tablespoon psyllium husk powder

2 teaspoons baking powder

½ teaspoon sea salt

4 tablespoons (½ stick) unsalted butter, at room temperature, plus more to grease the pan

1 tablespoon granulated erythritol–monk fruit blend

3½ ounces (about 7 tablespoons) cream cheese, at room temperature

4 large eggs, at room temperature

2 tablespoons sesame seeds

1. Preheat the oven to 350°F. Grease a 9-by-5-inch loaf pan with butter.

2. In a medium bowl, combine the almond flour, psyllium husk powder, baking powder, and salt. Set aside.

3. In a large bowl, using an electric mixer on medium-high speed, blend the butter and erythritol–monk fruit blend. Add the cream cheese, and combine well. Add the eggs one at a time, making sure to mix well after each addition. Add the dry ingredients to the wet ingredients, and mix well until the batter is fully combined.

4. Spread the batter in the prepared loaf pan, and sprinkle the sesame seeds on top. Bake the bread for 30 to 40 minutes, or until golden brown on top. The bread will be done when a toothpick inserted into the center comes out clean.

5. Allow to cool for about 10 minutes before removing from the pan. Place on a wire rack to cool for another 20 to 30 minutes to cool fully before slicing.

6. Store any leftovers in the refrigerator for up to 7 days, or freeze for up to 30 days. Toast the slices in a toaster or toaster oven.

Per serving: Calories: 165; Total Fat: 15g; Total Carbohydrates: 4g; Net Carbs: 2g; Fiber: 2g; Protein: 6g; Erythritol: 1g
Macros: Fat: 82%; Protein: 15%; Carbs: 3%

NUT-FREE SUNFLOWER BREAD

MAKES 12 SLICES / PREP TIME: 10 MINUTES / COOK TIME: 45 MINUTES TO 1 HOUR, PLUS 30 TO 40 MINUTES TO COOL
EQUIPMENT: 1 MIXING BOWL, ELECTRIC MIXER, 9-BY-5-INCH LOAF PAN

This sunflower bread is a tasty nut-free option. As an added plus, sunflower seed flour has 9.2 grams of polyunsaturated fat compared to 3.5 grams in almond flour, so it will keep you fuller longer. Delicious and satisfying, this recipe is a keto win.

Unsalted butter or coconut oil (to make the recipe dairy-free), for greasing the pan
1 cup coconut milk
½ cup coconut oil, melted and cooled
6 large eggs, at room temperature
1 cup sunflower seed flour

½ cup coconut flour
½ cup psyllium husk powder
½ cup granulated erythritol–monk fruit blend
1½ teaspoons baking powder
½ teaspoon sea salt
2 tablespoons sesame seeds

1. Preheat the oven to 350°F. Grease a 9-by-5-inch loaf pan with butter.

2. In a large bowl, using an electric mixer, combine the coconut milk and coconut oil. Add the eggs one at a time, mixing after each addition. Next, add the sunflower seed flour, coconut flour, psyllium husk powder, erythritol–monk fruit blend, baking powder, and salt. Mix the batter well on medium speed for about 2 minutes, or until fully incorporated. This batter will be thick.

3. Put the batter in the loaf pan. Sprinkle the sesame seeds on top. Bake for 45 minutes to 1 hour, or until a toothpick inserted into the center comes out clean.

4. Allow to cool for about 10 minutes before removing from the pan. Place on a wire rack for another 20 to 30 minutes to cool fully before slicing.

5. Store any leftovers in an airtight container in the refrigerator for up to 5 days, or freeze for up to 3 weeks.

Per serving: Calories: 233; Total Fat: 18g; Total Carbohydrates: 12g; Net Carbs: 4g; Fiber: 8g; Protein: 7g; Erythritol: 8g
Macros: Fat: 70%; Protein: 12%; Carbs: 18%

JALAPEÑO CHEESE BREAD

MAKES 12 SLICES / PREP TIME: 10 MINUTES / COOK TIME: 50 MINUTES TO 1 HOUR, PLUS 45 MINUTES TO COOL
EQUIPMENT: 2 MIXING BOWLS, COFFEE GRINDER, ELECTRIC MIXER, 9-BY-5-INCH LOAF PAN

With just a few essential ingredients from your keto pantry, you can make a simple, yummy, low-carb baked bread loaded with cheesy jalapeño goodness. Your taste buds and sugar levels will thank you for adding this classic flavor combination in keto-friendly form. Toast this bread and use it in a sandwich, or eat it as is. No matter how you slice it, this bread is made for eating.

4 tablespoons (¼ stick) unsalted butter, melted plus more to grease the pan
1 cup golden flax meal
¾ cup coconut flour
2 tablespoons granulated erythritol–monk fruit blend
3 tablespoons grated Parmesan cheese
1 tablespoon psyllium husk powder
2 teaspoons baking powder

1 teaspoon sea salt
¼ teaspoon black pepper
8 ounces (about 1 cup) cream cheese, softened
4 large eggs, at room temperature
3 cups shredded sharp Cheddar cheese, divided
⅓ cup pickled jalapeño peppers, diced
1¼ cups coconut milk or almond milk

1. Preheat the oven to 375°F. Grease a 9-by-5-inch loaf pan with butter, and line the bottom of the pan with parchment paper.

2. Grind the flax meal in a coffee grinder until it's a fine powder.

3. In a large bowl, combine the flax meal powder, coconut flour, erythritol–monk fruit blend, Parmesan cheese, psyllium husk powder, baking powder, salt, and pepper. Set aside.

4. In another large bowl, using an electric mixer on high speed, combine the cream cheese and eggs. Add 2 cups of Cheddar cheese and the pickled jalapeño peppers, and stir until well incorporated.

5. Add the dry ingredients to the wet ingredients, and combine well. Using a rubber spatula, fold in the melted butter. Add the coconut milk, and mix until just combined. The batter will be thick.

6. Spread the batter in the prepared loaf pan. Top with the remaining 1 cup of Cheddar cheese. Bake for 50 minutes to 1 hour or until the top is lightly browned and a toothpick inserted into the center comes out clean. Check the bread at the 45-minute mark, cover the top with aluminum foil to ensure it doesn't burn, and continue to bake until fully done.

7. Remove from the oven, and place on a wire rack. Allow to cool for at least 15 minutes before removing from the loaf pan. Allow to cool for another 30 minutes on a wire rack before slicing.

8. Store any leftovers in the refrigerator for up to 5 days, or freeze for up to 3 weeks.

Keep in Mind: Allow the parchment paper to overhang on the sides of the loaf pan so it's easy to remove the bread once baked. This also prevents the cheese from sticking to the bottom of the pan.

Per serving: Calories: 322; Total Fat: 26g; Total Carbohydrates: 12g; Net Carbs: 6g; Fiber: 6g; Protein: 13g; Erythritol: 2g
Macros: Fat: 73%; Protein: 16%; Carbs: 11%

BUTTERMILK BISCUITS

MAKES 10 BISCUITS / PREP TIME: 10 MINUTES / COOK TIME: 20 MINUTES
EQUIPMENT: 1 MIXING BOWL, LARGE BAKING SHEET

Now you can enjoy the tangy flavor of buttermilk biscuits without the high carbs of traditional biscuits. This recipe is tender and flaky and has a distinct buttermilk flavor without actually using any milk. The secret is a combination of sour cream, melted butter, and apple cider vinegar. These biscuits are sure to satisfy your craving for a Southern-style breakfast while keeping you in ketosis.

1¾ cups finely milled almond flour
2 tablespoons coconut flour
1 tablespoon baking powder
¼ teaspoon sea salt
½ cup sour cream

6 tablespoons unsalted butter,
  divided, melted
1 teaspoon apple cider vinegar
2 large eggs, at room temperature

1. Preheat the oven to 375°F. Line a large baking sheet with parchment paper or a silicone baking mat.

2. In a large bowl, measure then sift together the almond flour, coconut flour, baking powder, and salt. Add the sour cream, 4 tablespoons of melted butter, the apple cider vinegar, and eggs. Use a fork to combine until fully incorporated.

3. Drop the dough by large spoonfuls onto the baking sheet, and brush the tops of each biscuit with the remaining 2 tablespoons of melted butter. Bake the biscuits for 20 minutes, or until lightly golden brown on top. Serve hot or warm.

4. Store any leftovers in the refrigerator for up to 5 days, or freeze for up to 3 weeks.

Per serving: Calories: 203; Total Fat: 18g; Total Carbohydrates: 7g; Net Carbs: 4g; Fiber: 3g; Protein: 6g; Erythritol: 0g
Macros: Fat: 80%; Protein: 12%; Carbs: 8%

CHEDDAR-CHIVE BISCUITS

MAKES 10 BISCUITS / PREP TIME: 10 MINUTES / COOK TIME: 20 MINUTES
EQUIPMENT: 1 MIXING BOWL, LARGE BAKING SHEET

One bite of these melt-in-your-mouth biscuits will have you convinced that this keto diet thing can indeed be delicious. The recipe uses a combination of almond flour, coconut flour, and sour cream to produce the perfect fluffy, low-carb biscuits. Why should you be craving a traditional biscuit when you can have a tender keto one in about half an hour?

1¾ cup finely milled almond flour
2 tablespoons coconut flour
1 tablespoon baking powder
¼ teaspoon sea salt
½ cup sour cream
½ cup shredded sharp Cheddar cheese

4 tablespoons (¼ stick) unsalted butter, melted, plus more for serving
2 large eggs, at room temperature
2 tablespoons finely chopped chives
2 tablespoons grated Parmesan cheese

1. Preheat the oven to 375°F. Line a large baking sheet with parchment paper or a silicone baking mat.

2. In a large bowl, measure then sift together the almond flour, coconut flour, baking powder, and salt. Add the sour cream, Cheddar cheese, melted butter, eggs, and chives. Use a fork to combine until fully incorporated.

3. Drop the dough by large spoonfuls onto the baking sheet, and sprinkle the top of each biscuit with Parmesan cheese. Bake the biscuits for 20 minutes, or until lightly golden brown on top. Serve your biscuits hot from the oven with butter.

4. Store any leftovers in the refrigerator for up to 5 days, or freeze for up to 3 weeks.

Variation Tip: You can replace the Cheddar cheese and chives with pepper jack cheese for a spiced-up version of this classic.

Per serving: Calories: 229; Total Fat: 20g; Total Carbohydrates: 7g; Net Carbs: 4g; Fiber: 3g; Protein: 8g; Erythritol: 0g
Macros: Fat: 79%; Protein: 14%; Carbs: 7%

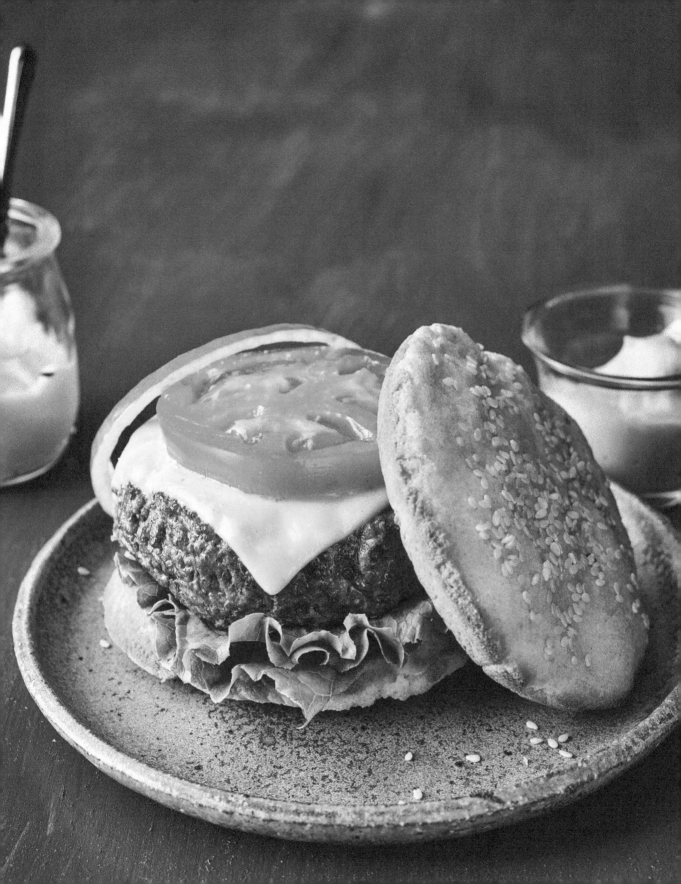

SESAME BURGER BUNS

MAKES 9 BUNS / PREP TIME: 10 MINUTES / COOK TIME: 50 MINUTES TO 1 HOUR, PLUS 20 MINUTES TO COOL
EQUIPMENT: 2 MIXING BOWLS, ELECTRIC MIXER, 12-CUP MUFFIN TOP PAN OR LARGE BAKING SHEET

Lettuce-wrapped burgers are okay, but sometimes you are in the mood to pick up a burger with your hands and not worry about it spilling all over the place. I'm here to tell you that this simple burger bun recipe will satisfy this need without sacrificing flavor or putting your keto success in jeopardy. This recipe has you use a muffin top pan, which has wider, shallower cups than a regular muffin pan. I like to use the Wilton Perfect Results premium nonstick muffin top baking pan to get consistent perfect-size buns.

4 tablespoons (½ stick) unsalted butter, at room temperature, plus more for greasing the pan

¾ cup coconut flour

1 tablespoon psyllium husk powder

2 teaspoons baking powder

1 teaspoon granulated erythritol–monk fruit blend

½ teaspoon sea salt

4 ounces (about ½ cup) cream cheese, at room temperature

4 large eggs, at room temperature

¼ cup full-fat sour cream

2 tablespoons salted butter, melted

1 tablespoon sesame seeds

1. Preheat the oven to 350°F. Generously grease a 12-cup muffin top pan with butter.

2. In a medium bowl, combine the coconut flour, psyllium husk powder, baking powder, erythritol–monk fruit blend, and salt.

3. In a large bowl, using an electric mixer, beat the butter and cream cheese until light and fluffy. Scrape down the sides of the bowl several times with a rubber spatula to make sure the mixture is well blended. Add the eggs one at a time, mixing after each addition.

4. Add the dry ingredients to the wet ingredients slowly while mixing on low speed. Make sure to scrape down the bowl a couple of times. When the two mixtures are fully combined, gently fold in the sour cream. Make sure the sour cream gets fully incorporated into the batter, but be careful to not overmix.

Continued →

5. Overfill the cups of the muffin top pan just slightly with batter. The batter should be thick and fluffy (normal for batter made with coconut flour) so the buns will not spread too much when baked. Brush the top of each muffin top with the melted butter and then sprinkle the sesame seeds on top of 9 of the buns. Bake the buns for 25 to 30 minutes, or until lightly browned on the top and a toothpick inserted into the center comes out clean.

6. Allow the buns to cool for 10 minutes in the pan before removing.

7. You will have enough leftover batter to fill 6 more muffin top cups. Once the pan has cooled, regrease the 6 openings, and bake the additional 6 buns. This will yield a total of 9 top and 9 bottom burger buns. Use the muffin tops that do not have sesame seeds as your bottom buns and the ones with sesame seeds as your tops.

8. Store any leftovers in the refrigerator for up to 5 days, or freeze for up to 3 weeks.

Keep in Mind: If you don't have (or don't want to buy) a muffin top pan, you can just spoon burger bun–size circles of the batter onto a greased baking sheet, and bake.

Per serving: Calories: 209; Total Fat: 17g; Total Carbohydrates: 9g; Net Carbs: 4g; Fiber: 5g; Protein: 6g; Erythritol: <1g
Macros: Fat: 73%; Protein: 11%; Carbs: 16%

CHEESY GARLIC ROLLS

MAKES 12 ROLLS / PREP TIME: 10 MINUTES / COOK TIME: 25 TO 30 MINUTES
EQUIPMENT: 2 MIXING BOWLS, LARGE BAKING SHEET

There is nothing like the smell of fresh-baked cheesy garlic rolls to bring the family running to the kitchen. With just a few key ingredients, you can make a keto-friendly side dish that you can gladly say yes to.

1½ cups shredded mozzarella cheese
¼ cup cream cheese, at room temperature
2 large eggs, at room temperature
¾ cup finely milled almond flour, measured and sifted

3 tablespoons salted butter
1 teaspoon extra-virgin olive oil
2 cloves garlic, minced
¼ teaspoon garlic salt
¼ cup grated Parmesan cheese
¼ cup chopped fresh flat-leaf parsley

1. Preheat the oven to 350°F. Line a large baking sheet with parchment paper.

2. Put the mozzarella cheese in a medium microwave-safe bowl. Microwave in 30-second increments, making sure to stir each time, until fully melted. Add the cream cheese, and combine well. Allow the mixture to cool slightly and then stir in the eggs and almond flour. The dough will be sticky.

3. Using wet hands, separate the dough into 12 equal parts and shape into rounds. Place them on the prepared baking sheet.

4. In a small bowl, to make the garlic butter, combine the butter, olive oil, garlic, and garlic salt. With a pastry brush, spread the garlic butter on top of each roll, and sprinkle with the Parmesan cheese.

5. Bake for 25 to 30 minutes, or until lightly golden. Top with the parsley right out of the oven. Serve hot or warm.

6. Store any leftovers in an airtight container in the refrigerator for up to 3 days.

Per serving: Calories: 148; Total Fat: 12g; Total Carbohydrates: 3g; Net Carbs: 2g; Fiber: 1g; Protein: 7g; Erythritol: 0g
Macros: Fat: 73%; Protein: 19%; Carbs: 8%

SAVORY NAAN

MAKES 6 NAAN / PREP TIME: 10 MINUTES / COOK TIME: 15 TO 20 MINUTES, PLUS COOLING TIME
EQUIPMENT: 1 MIXING BOWL, COFFEE GRINDER, LARGE BAKING SHEET

It's hard to believe that this soft and doughy naan is low in carbs and keto-friendly, and yet it is. The best part of this bread is how very easy it is to make. Serve alongside your favorite keto-friendly curries, or spread with your favorite toppings to make a pizza. You simply can't go wrong with this naan.

1½ tablespoons golden flax meal

1½ cups finely milled almond flour, measured and sifted

2 teaspoons psyllium husk powder

2 teaspoons sesame seeds

2 teaspoons baking powder

½ teaspoon onion powder

½ teaspoon garlic powder

¼ teaspoon xanthan gum

¼ teaspoon sea salt

1 cup hot water

1 teaspoon extra-virgin olive oil

2 large eggs, at room temperature

1 tablespoon salted butter, melted

2 tablespoons fresh flat-leaf parsley, chopped

2 teaspoons sea salt flakes

1. Preheat the oven to 375°F. Line a large baking sheet with a silicone baking mat or parchment paper.

2. In a coffee grinder, grind the flax meal until it's a fine powder.

3. In a large bowl, combine the flax meal powder, almond flour, psyllium husk powder, sesame seeds, baking powder, onion powder, garlic powder, xanthan gum, and salt. Add the hot water, olive oil, and eggs. Mix the dough well with a silicone spatula.

4. Scoop 6 equal portions of the dough onto the prepared baking sheet. With wet hands, form them into circles. Be sure to keep your hands wet because the dough will be very sticky.

5. Using a pastry brush, brush each naan with the melted butter. Sprinkle the tops of the naans evenly with the parsley and sea salt flakes.

6. Bake for 15 to 20 minutes, or until lightly browned.

7. Allow to cool slightly on the baking sheet before serving.

8. Store any leftovers in the refrigerator for up to 5 days, or freeze for up to 3 weeks.

Variation Tip: To easily make this dairy-free, replace the butter with melted coconut oil.

Per serving: Calories: 227; Total Fat: 19g; Total Carbohydrates: 9g; Net Carbs: 4g; Fiber: 5g; Protein: 9g; Erythritol: 0g
Macros: Fat: 75%; Protein: 16%; Carbs: 9%

ONION-GARLIC PITA BREAD

MAKES 6 PITAS / PREP TIME: 10 MINUTES / COOK TIME: 25 TO 35 MINUTES, PLUS COOLING TIME
EQUIPMENT: 1 MIXING BOWL, COFFEE GRINDER, LARGE BAKING SHEET

Full of flavor, this pita bread recipe is made with a combination of almond flour, golden flax meal, and psyllium husk powder. This pita recipe will not produce a pocket like traditional pita bread, because of the lack of gluten. However, they are quite bendy, which allows you to fold them and add your favorite fillings.

3 tablespoons golden flax meal

3 cups finely milled almond flour, measured and sifted

1 tablespoon psyllium husk powder

2 teaspoons sesame seeds

2 teaspoons baking powder

½ teaspoon xanthan gum

½ teaspoon sea salt

½ teaspoon onion powder

½ teaspoon garlic powder

1 cup hot water

1 tablespoon extra-virgin olive oil or melted coconut oil

2 large eggs, at room temperature

1 tablespoon salted butter, melted

¼ chopped parsley

Sea salt flakes

1. Preheat the oven to 400°F. Line a large baking sheet with a silicone baking mat or parchment paper.

2. In a coffee grinder, grind the flax meal until it's a fine powder.

3. In a large bowl, combine the flax meal powder, almond flour, psyllium husk powder, sesame seeds, baking powder, xanthan gum, salt, onion powder, and garlic powder. Add the hot water, olive oil, and eggs. Mix the dough well with a silicone spatula.

4. Scoop 6 equal portions of the dough onto the prepared baking sheet. With wet hands, form them into circles. Be sure to keep your hands wet because the dough will be very sticky.

5. Using a pastry brush, brush each pita with the melted butter. Sprinkle the tops of the breads evenly with the fresh parsley and sea salt flakes.

6. Bake for 25 to 35 minutes, or until lightly browned.

7. Allow to cool fully on the baking sheet before serving.

8. Store any leftovers in the refrigerator for up to 5 days, or freeze for up to 3 weeks.

Keep in Mind: It's important not to overbake the pita bread and to cook only until lightly browned, so that they remain flexible enough to use as sandwich bread.

Per serving: Calories: 409; Total Fat: 36g; Total Carbohydrates: 15g; Net Carbs: 7g; Fiber: 8g; Protein: 15g; Erythritol: 2g
Macros: Fat: 79%; Protein: 15%; Carbs: 6%

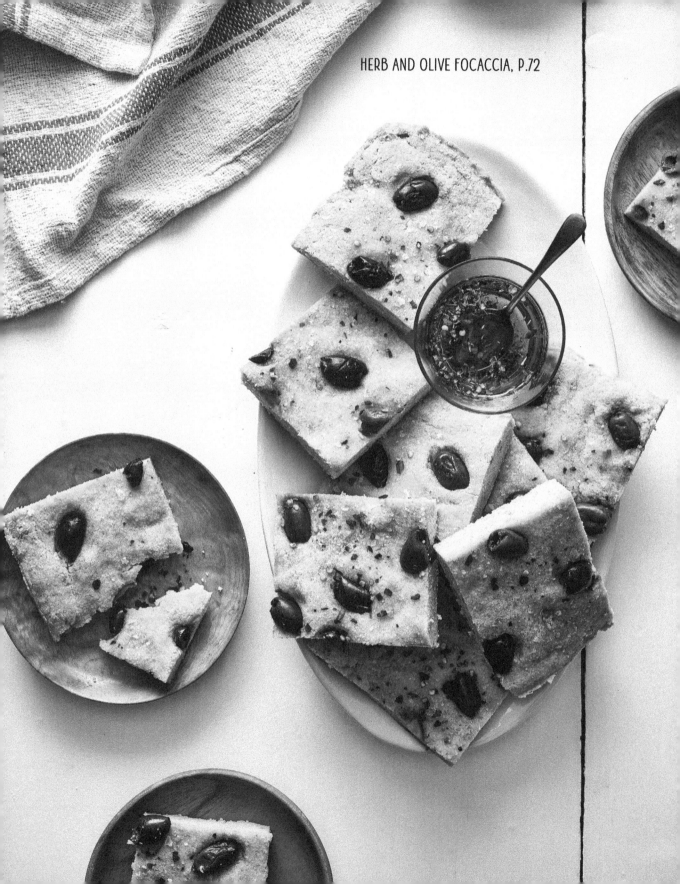

HERB AND OLIVE FOCACCIA, P.72

CHAPTER 5

FLATBREADS, PIZZAS, AND SPECIALTY BREADS

ROSEMARY FLATBREAD

MAKES 6 FLATBREADS / PREP TIME: 10 MINUTES / COOK TIME: 25 TO 35 MINUTES
EQUIPMENT: 1 MIXING BOWL, COFFEE GRINDER, LARGE BAKING SHEET

The basis of any great flatbread is the dough, and this rosemary-infused flatbread works beautifully despite the lack of gluten. With just a few key ingredients, you can enjoy a perfect keto option that can be served as an appetizer or as bread alongside a keto meal. The best part is that this recipe comes together quickly, allowing you to enjoy it fast and often.

1½ tablespoons golden flax meal
1½ cups finely milled almond flour, measured and sifted
2 teaspoons psyllium husk powder
1 teaspoon baking powder
¼ teaspoon xanthan gum
¼ teaspoon sea salt
¼ teaspoon onion powder

¼ teaspoon garlic powder
½ cup hot water
1 tablespoon extra-virgin olive oil, plus more for brushing
1 large egg, at room temperature
1½ tablespoons chopped fresh rosemary
Sea salt flakes

1. Preheat the oven to 400°F. Line a large baking sheet with a silicone baking mat or parchment paper.

2. In a coffee grinder, grind the flax meal until it's a fine powder.

3. In a large bowl, combine the flax meal powder, almond flour, psyllium husk powder, baking powder, xanthan gum, salt, onion powder, and garlic powder. Add the hot water, olive oil, and egg. Mix the dough well with a silicone spatula.

4. Scoop 6 equal portions of the dough onto the baking sheet. With wet hands, form the dough into circles. Be sure to keep your hands wet because the dough will be very sticky.

5. Use a pastry brush to brush each flatbread with olive oil. Sprinkle the tops evenly with the rosemary and sea salt flakes. Bake for 25 to 35 minutes, or until lightly browned.

6. Serve this flatbread straight from the oven. No cooling necessary.

7. Store any leftovers in the refrigerator for up to 5 days, or freeze for up to 3 weeks.

Variation Tip: You can use this flatbread to make personal pizzas by simply topping it with your favorite low-sugar pizza sauce and keto-friendly toppings.

Per serving: Calories: 225; Total Fat: 20g; Total Carbohydrates: 8g; Net Carbs: 4g; Fiber: 4g; Protein: 8g; Erythritol: 0g
Macros: Fat: 80%; Protein: 14%; Carbs: 6%

HERB AND OLIVE FOCACCIA

MAKES 10 SQUARES / PREP TIME: 10 MINUTES / COOK TIME: 25 TO 35 MINUTES
EQUIPMENT: 1 MIXING BOWL, COFFEE GRINDER, LARGE BAKING SHEET

Before my keto days, my favorite places to dine out were Italian restaurants, mostly for the bread and oil at the beginning. I thought this was something I wouldn't be able to enjoy ever again with my new keto lifestyle. With my focus originally mainly on creating keto desserts, I didn't create a perfect duplicate for my favorite until recently (I know—how could I forget a favorite?!). I'm here to tell you that you can enjoy my (and probably your) favorite part of Italian dining out and stay within your macros! This focaccia and bread dipping oil comes together so quickly and easily that it will become a staple in your home in no time.

FOR THE BREAD

3 tablespoons golden flax meal

3 cups finely milled almond flour, measured and sifted

1 tablespoon psyllium husk powder

2 teaspoons baking powder

½ teaspoon xanthan gum

½ teaspoon sea salt

½ teaspoon onion powder

½ teaspoon garlic powder

1 cup hot water

3 tablespoons extra-virgin olive oil, divided

2 large eggs, at room temperature

20 Kalamata olives, pitted

2 teaspoons sea salt flakes

¼ teaspoon red pepper flakes

FOR THE BREAD DIPPING OIL

½ cup extra-virgin olive oil

1 tablespoon sea salt

1 tablespoon dried oregano

1 tablespoon dried rosemary

2 teaspoons freshly ground pepper

2 teaspoons red pepper flakes

TO MAKE THE BREAD

1. Preheat the oven to 400°F. Line a large baking sheet with a silicone baking mat or parchment paper.

2. In a coffee grinder, grind the flax meal until it's a fine powder.

3. In a large bowl, combine the flax meal powder, almond flour, psyllium husk powder, baking powder, xanthan gum, salt, onion powder, and garlic powder. Add the hot water, 1 tablespoon of extra-virgin olive oil, and eggs. Mix the dough well with a silicone spatula.

4. With wet hands, spread the dough evenly over the baking sheet. Using a pastry brush, spread the remaining 2 tablespoons of olive oil over the entire surface of the dough. Sprinkle the olives, sea salt flakes, and red pepper flakes over the top. Lightly press the olives into the dough. Bake for 25 to 35 minutes, or until lightly browned.

TO MAKE THE BREAD DIPPING OIL AND FINISH THE BREAD

1. While the bread is baking, combine the olive oil, salt, oregano, rosemary, pepper, and red pepper flakes in a small bowl.

2. Remove the bread from the oven, and cut into 10 squares. Enjoy while still warm with the dipping oil.

3. Store any leftover bread in the refrigerator for up to 5 days, or freeze for up to 3 weeks. Store any leftover dipping oil in a sealed container in a cool, dry place for up to 2 days.

Variation Tip: You can customize this focaccia any way you like by substituting your favorite toppings, herbs, and spices. For example, instead of olives, you could use halved cherry tomatoes for a roasted tomato and herb focaccia if that fits with your macros.

Per serving: Calories: 375; Total Fat: 36g; Total Carbohydrates: 10g; Net Carbs: 5g; Fiber: 5g; Protein: 9g; Erythritol: 0g
Macros: Fat: 86%; Protein: 10%; Carbs: 4%

BLACKBERRY, PROSCIUTTO, AND GOAT CHEESE FLATBREAD

MAKES 6 FLATBREADS / PREP TIME: 15 MINUTES / COOK TIME: 40 TO 50 MINUTES, PLUS COOLING TIME
EQUIPMENT: 2 MIXING BOWLS, COFFEE GRINDER, LARGE BAKING SHEET

This mouthwatering blackberry flatbread appetizer combines the rich textures and flavors of prosciutto, berries, and goat cheese for a bold and elevated dish. The sweet-to-salty ratio in this flatbread is pure perfection, but you can also swap out the goat cheese spread for fresh burrata and the blackberries for whole raspberries for another flavor profile. Share this with your guests during your next get-together, and let them taste firsthand how decadent the keto diet can be.

FOR THE FLATBREAD

3 tablespoons golden flax meal
3 cups finely milled almond flour, measured and sifted
1 tablespoon psyllium husk powder
2 teaspoons baking powder
½ teaspoon xanthan gum
½ teaspoon sea salt
¼ teaspoon onion powder
¼ teaspoon garlic powder
1 cup hot water
1 tablespoon extra-virgin olive oil
2 large eggs, at room temperature

FOR THE TOPPINGS

1 cup crumbled goat cheese, at room temperature, divided
¼ cup heavy whipping cream
2 tablespoons cream cheese, at room temperature
2 tablespoons unsalted butter, melted
½ pint fresh blackberries, quartered
½ cup fresh basil, chiffonade
6 slices prosciutto, torn into small pieces
1 tablespoon balsamic vinegar

TO MAKE THE FLATBREAD

1. Preheat the oven to 400°F. Line a large baking sheet with a silicone baking mat or parchment paper.

2. In a coffee grinder, grind the flax meal until it's a fine powder.

3. In a large bowl, combine the flax meal powder, almond flour, psyllium husk powder, baking powder, xanthan gum, salt, onion powder, and garlic powder. Add the hot water, olive oil, and eggs. Mix the dough well with a silicone spatula.

4. Scoop 6 equal portions of the dough onto the baking sheet. With wet hands, form the dough into circles. Be sure to keep your hands wet because the dough will be very sticky.

5. Bake for 25 to 35 minutes, or until lightly browned.

6. Allow to cool completely on the baking sheet before topping.

TO MAKE THE TOPPINGS AND FINISH THE FLATBREAD

1. In a small bowl, combine ¾ cup of goat cheese, the heavy whipping cream, and cream cheese.

2. Once the flatbreads have fully cooled, use a pastry brush to baste each flatbread with the melted butter. Spread the goat cheese mixture evenly on top, and top with the blackberries, basil, prosciutto, and remaining ¼ cup of goat cheese.

3. Bake for another 15 minutes, or until the goat cheese has melted and slightly browned. Drizzle with the balsamic vinegar right before serving.

4. Store any leftovers in the refrigerator for up to 3 days.

Ingredient tip: To chiffonade basil, stack 5 to 6 basil leaves on top of each other, roll them together into a cigar-like shape, then use a sharp knife to thinly slice into ribbons. Stacking too many together will make it harder to cut through, so do this in batches if you need to chiffonade a lot of basil.

Per serving: Calories: 574; Total Fat: 49g; Total Carbohydrates: 20g; Net Carbs: 10g; Fiber: 10g; Protein: 22g; Erythritol: 0g
Macros: Fat: 77%; Protein: 15%; Carbs: 8%

PEPPERONI SUPREME PIZZA

MAKES 1 (14-INCH) PIZZA (8 SLICES) / PREP TIME: 15 MINUTES / COOK TIME: 30 TO 40 MINUTES
EQUIPMENT: 2 MIXING BOWLS, MEDIUM SAUCEPAN, 14-INCH PIZZA PAN

I've always been a big fan of pizza and have tried every kind of keto pizza out there. Trust me: This delicious keto-friendly supreme pizza tastes like the real deal. The crust uses a mozzarella dough that I have customized to give it more of a bread-like texture. Obviously, you can change up the toppings as you like. And if you don't have a round pizza pan, you can use a parchment paper–lined large baking sheet.

FOR THE SAUCE
2 tablespoons extra-virgin olive oil
2 cloves garlic, crushed
1 (14-ounce) can crushed tomatoes
1 teaspoon Italian seasoning
1 teaspoon dried basil
1 teaspoon dried oregano
1 teaspoon sea salt
¼ teaspoon red pepper flakes

FOR THE CRUST
Extra-virgin olive oil, for
    greasing the pan
3 cups shredded mozzarella cheese
2 tablespoons cream cheese
2 large eggs, at room temperature
1¼ cups finely milled almond flour,
    measured and sifted
¼ cup coconut flour

FOR THE TOPPINGS
1 cup shredded mozzarella cheese
¼ cup sliced pepperoni
¼ cup chopped onions
¼ cup chopped green bell pepper
¼ cup sliced mushrooms
¼ cup sliced black olives
¼ cup grated Parmesan cheese

TO MAKE THE SAUCE
1. Heat the olive oil in a medium saucepan over medium-high heat. Sauté the garlic until translucent. Add the crushed tomatoes, Italian seasoning, basil, oregano, salt, and red pepper flakes.

2. Lower the heat to a simmer, and cook the sauce until it has reduced and thickened, for about 15 minutes. Set aside.

TO MAKE THE CRUST

1. Preheat the oven to 375°F. Lightly grease a 14-inch pizza pan with olive oil.

2. Put the mozzarella cheese in a medium microwave-safe bowl. Microwave in 30-second increments, making sure to stir each time, until fully melted. Add the cream cheese to the melted mozzarella, and combine well. Allow the mixture to cool slightly and then stir in the eggs, almond flour, and coconut flour.

3. Using wet hands, press the dough into the pizza pan, and stretch to cover it. Pierce the surface of the pizza crust all over with a fork.

4. Bake for 10 minutes, then check for any large bubbles that may have formed, and poke with a fork to deflate them. Continue baking for another 5 to 10 minutes, or until golden brown on top. Take the pan out of the oven, and allow to cool for at least 15 minutes.

TO MAKE THE TOPPINGS AND FINISH THE PIZZA

1. Spread the sauce evenly over the crust, and sprinkle the mozzarella cheese on top.

2. Add the pepperoni, onions, bell pepper, mushrooms, olives, and Parmesan cheese, and bake for another 15 to 20 minutes, or until all the toppings are cooked and the cheese is slightly browned around the edges. Serve hot.

3. Store any leftovers wrapped in plastic wrap or in an airtight container in the refrigerator for up to 3 days.

Keep in Mind: Piercing the dough with a fork before baking is important to help reduce air pockets while the crust cooks.

Per serving: Calories: 384; Total Fat: 28g; Total Carbohydrates: 12g; Net Carbs: 8g; Fiber: 4g; Protein: 25g; Erythritol: 0g
Macros: Fat: 66%; Protein: 26%; Carbs: 8%

BACON AND EGG PIZZA

MAKES 1 (14-INCH) PIZZA (8 SLICES) / PREP TIME: 15 MINUTES / COOK TIME: 30 TO 40 MINUTES
EQUIPMENT: 1 MIXING BOWL, 14-INCH PIZZA PAN

Who says you can't eat pizza in the morning? For that matter, who says you can't eat bacon and eggs for dinner? I tweaked the famous mozzarella dough we all love so that it holds bacon and eggs beautifully. This pizza makes the keto diet a delicious breeze when mornings start with pizza. If you don't have a round pizza pan, you can use a large parchment paper–lined baking sheet.

FOR THE CRUST
Extra-virgin olive oil, for
    greasing the pan
3 cups shredded mozzarella cheese
¼ cup cream cheese
2 large eggs, at room temperature
1¼ cups finely milled almond flour,
    measured and sifted
¼ cup coconut flour

FOR THE TOPPINGS
1 tablespoon extra-virgin olive oil
1 cup shredded mozzarella cheese
5 slices cooked bacon, crumbled
4 large eggs, at room temperature
2 tablespoons grated Parmesan cheese
2 tablespoons minced chives

TO MAKE THE CRUST

1. Preheat the oven to 375°F. Lightly grease a 14-inch pizza pan with olive oil.

2. Put the mozzarella cheese in a medium microwave-safe bowl. Microwave in 30-second increments, making sure to stir each time, until fully melted. Add the cream cheese to the melted mozzarella, and combine well. Allow the mixture to cool slightly and then stir in the eggs, almond flour, and coconut flour.

3. Using wet hands, press the dough into the pizza pan, and stretch to cover it. Pierce the surface of the pizza crust all over with a fork.

4. Bake for 10 minutes, then check for any large bubbles that may have formed, and poke with a fork to deflate them. Continue baking for another 5 to 10 minutes, or until golden brown on top. Take the pan out of the oven, and allow to cool for at least 15 minutes.

TO MAKE THE TOPPINGS AND FINISH THE PIZZA

1. Spread the olive oil evenly over the crust. Sprinkle on the mozzarella cheese, then the bacon. Carefully crack the eggs on the top, spacing them evenly. Sprinkle on the Parmesan cheese.

2. Bake for 15 to 20 minutes, or until the eggs are cooked. Garnish with the chives, then cut and serve hot.

3. Store any leftovers wrapped in plastic wrap or in an airtight container in the refrigerator for 1 day.

Keep in Mind: Be careful not to overcook the eggs; you'll want the egg yolk to be set but slightly runny.

Per serving: Calories: 401; Total Fat: 29g; Total Carbohydrates: 9g; Net Carbs: 6g; Fiber: 3g; Protein: 28g; Erythritol: 0g
Macros: Fat: 65%; Protein: 28%; Carbs: 7%

GOAT CHEESE AND BASIL PIZZA

MAKES 1 (14-INCH) PIZZA (8 SLICES) / PREP TIME: 15 MINUTES / COOK TIME: 30 TO 40 MINUTES, PLUS 15 MINUTES TO COOL
EQUIPMENT: 2 MIXING BOWLS, MEDIUM SAUCEPAN, 14-INCH PIZZA PAN

This pizza starts by using my perfected keto pizza dough and topping it with goat cheese and basil to create a Mediterranean-style pizza. The tangy, creamy goat cheese pairs beautifully with the mild sweetness from the basil to give you a light and flavorful pizza.

FOR THE SAUCE
2 tablespoons extra-virgin olive oil
2 cloves garlic, crushed
1 (14-ounce) can crushed tomatoes
1 teaspoon Italian seasoning
1 teaspoon dried basil
1 teaspoon dried oregano
1 teaspoon sea salt
¼ teaspoon red pepper flakes

FOR THE CRUST
Extra-virgin olive oil, for
    greasing the pan
3 cups shredded mozzarella cheese
¼ cup cream cheese
2 large eggs, at room temperature
1¼ cups finely milled almond flour,
    measured and sifted
¼ cup coconut flour

FOR THE TOPPINGS
1 cup crumbled goat cheese
½ cup fresh basil, chiffonade
2 teaspoons minced fresh rosemary

TO MAKE THE SAUCE
1. Heat the olive oil in a medium saucepan over medium-high heat. Sauté the garlic until translucent. Add the crushed tomatoes, Italian seasoning, basil, oregano, salt, and red pepper flakes.

2. Lower the heat to a simmer, and cook the sauce until it has reduced and thickened, for about 15 minutes. Set aside.

TO MAKE THE CRUST

1. Preheat the oven to 375°F. Lightly grease a 14-inch pizza pan with olive oil.

2. Put the mozzarella cheese in a medium microwave-safe bowl. Microwave in 30-second increments, making sure to stir each time, until fully melted. Add the cream cheese to the melted mozzarella, and combine well. Allow the mixture to cool slightly and then stir in the eggs, almond flour, and coconut flour.

3. Using wet hands, press the dough into the pizza pan, and stretch to cover it. Pierce the surface of the pizza crust all over with a fork.

4. Bake for 10 minutes, then check for any large bubbles that may have formed, and poke with a fork to deflate them. Continue baking for another 5 to 10 minutes, or until golden brown on top. Take the pan out of the oven, and allow to cool for at least 15 minutes.

TO MAKE THE TOPPINGS AND FINISH THE PIZZA

1. Spread the sauce evenly over the crust, and sprinkle the goat cheese on top. Add the basil and rosemary. Bake for another 15 to 20 minutes, or until the cheese is melted.

2. Store any leftovers wrapped in plastic wrap or in an airtight container in the refrigerator for up to 3 days.

Variation Tip: For a more classic Margherita pizza, substitute fresh, full-fat mozzarella for the goat cheese, omit the rosemary, and add some diced tomatoes.

Per serving: Calories: 356; Total Fat: 27g; Total Carbohydrates: 10g; Net Carbs: 6g; Fiber: 4g; Protein: 22g; Erythritol: 0g
Macros: Fat: 68%; Protein: 25%; Carbs: 7%

FLAX MEAL TORTILLAS

MAKES 8 TORTILLAS / PREP TIME: 10 MINUTES, PLUS RESTING TIME / COOK TIME: 10 MINUTES
EQUIPMENT: 1 MIXING BOWL, COFFEE GRINDER, LARGE NONSTICK SKILLET

These flax tortillas are tender, soft, and flexible. They also happen to be super easy to make. Whether eaten alone or filled, these tortillas will allow you to enjoy a low-carb option that is not only delicious but also full of nutrition and fiber. They are sure to become part of your keto taco Tuesdays.

¾ cup golden flax meal
¼ cup coconut flour
1 tablespoon psyllium husk powder
½ teaspoon xanthan gum

½ teaspoon sea salt
1 cup hot water
1 tablespoon coconut or olive oil

1. In a coffee grinder, grind the flax meal until it's a fine powder.

2. In a large bowl, combine the flax meal powder, coconut flour, psyllium husk powder, xanthan gum, and salt. Add the hot water and olive oil.

3. Mix the dough well with a silicone spatula. Then allow the dough to rest, covered with a kitchen towel, for about 10 minutes.

4. Use your hands to form the dough into 8 equal balls. Flatten each ball between 2 sheets of parchment paper or a tortilla press to form 8 (5-inch) tortillas.

5. In a large nonstick skillet over medium heat, cook each tortilla for about 10 to 15 seconds and then flip. Cook until both sides are golden, for 20 to 30 seconds total. Keep your tortillas warm by wrapping them in a kitchen towel. Serve immediately.

6. Store any leftovers in the refrigerator for up to 5 days, or freeze for up to 3 weeks. To warm, simply reheat in the skillet until just warm.

Variation Tip: For an extra punch of flavor, you can add 1 tablespoon of onion flakes when you add the salt.

Per serving: Calories: 79; Total Fat: 6g; Total Carbohydrates: 7g; Net Carbs: 2g; Fiber: 5g; Protein: 3g; Erythritol: 0g
Macros: Fat: 68%; Protein: 15%; Carbs: 17%

SESAME SEED CRACKERS

MAKES 20 CRACKERS / PREP TIME: 15 MINUTES / COOK TIME: 50 MINUTES TO 1 HOUR, PLUS COOLING TIME
EQUIPMENT: 1 MIXING BOWL, LARGE BAKING SHEET

Deliciously crispy, these sesame seed crackers are packed with spices and cheesy flavor. The dough for these crackers is straightforward and comes together quickly. Then it's just a matter of rolling the dough thinly between parchment paper, slicing, and baking. These crackers can be enjoyed as is or used to scoop up your favorite keto-friendly dips.

½ cup shredded sharp Cheddar cheese
½ cup finely grated shelf-stable Parmesan cheese
½ cup grated Parmesan cheese
½ cup coconut flour
½ cup sesame seeds
2 teaspoons psyllium husk powder
1 teaspoon baking powder
1 teaspoon onion powder
1 teaspoon garlic powder
1 teaspoon dried basil

1 teaspoon dried oregano
½ teaspoon sea salt
¼ teaspoon freshly ground black pepper
¼ teaspoon red pepper flakes
1 cup water
3 tablespoons avocado oil or extra-virgin olive oil
1 large egg, at room temperature
2 tablespoons white sesame seeds
2 tablespoons black sesame seeds

1. Preheat the oven to 350°F. Line a large baking sheet with parchment paper.

2. In a large mixing bowl, combine the Cheddar cheese, shelf-stable Parmesan cheese, Parmesan cheese, coconut flour, sesame seeds, psyllium husk powder, baking powder, onion powder, garlic powder, basil, oregano, salt, pepper, and red pepper flakes. Stir until well combined. Add the water, oil, and egg, and stir until a smooth dough forms.

3. Divide the dough in half, and roll one half out thinly between 2 sheets of parchment paper. The thinner you roll out the dough, the crispier the crackers.

4. Using a pizza cutter, cut the dough into crackers, and carefully place on a parchment paper–lined baking sheet (you may need to transfer them using a pancake spatula). Sprinkle the black and white sesame seeds on top of the crackers.

Continued →

5. Bake for 25 to 30 minutes, or until lightly browned around the edges.

6. Repeat with the other half of the dough.

7. Allow to cool fully in the baking sheet before serving.

8. Store any leftovers in the refrigerator for up to 5 days, or freeze for up to 3 weeks.

Keep in Mind: You can opt for a more organic shape and bake the whole cracker dough on 2 baking sheets. Once they are baked and cooled, you can break them into pieces.

Per serving: Calories: 94; Total Fat: 7g; Total Carbohydrates: 4g; Net Carbs: 2g; Fiber: 2g; Protein: 4g; Erythritol: 0g
Macros: Fat: 67%; Protein: 17%; Carbs: 16%

SOFT-BAKED PRETZELS WITH SPICY MUSTARD DIP

MAKES 10 PRETZELS / PREP TIME: 20 MINUTES, PLUS RISING TIME / COOK TIME: 25 TO 30 MINUTES, PLUS COOLING TIME
EQUIPMENT: 4 MIXING BOWLS, LARGE BAKING SHEET

Soft, chewy, and full of flavor, this recipe will singlehandedly bring back memories of indulging in warm, soft-baked pretzels at a fair or sporting event. I also included my recipe for a spicy mustard dipping sauce, making this the perfect combination for a game-day snack.

FOR THE SPICY MUSTARD DIP
¼ cup full-fat mayonnaise
¼ cup prepared yellow mustard
1½ teaspoons prepared horseradish
1 teaspoon Tabasco sauce
½ teaspoon sea salt
½ teaspoon onion powder
¼ teaspoon red pepper flakes
¼ teaspoon freshly ground
   black pepper
¼ teaspoon garlic powder

FOR THE PRETZELS
1 tablespoon yeast
1 teaspoon inulin fiber or sugar
3 tablespoons warm water
2 cups shredded part-skim mozzarella
   cheese, melted
2 tablespoons cream cheese, at room
   temperature
¾ cup coconut flour
2 teaspoons baking powder
¼ teaspoon xanthan gum
2 large eggs, at room temperature
1 large egg white, at room temperature
Coarse sea salt

TO MAKE THE SPICY MUSTARD DIP
1. In a medium bowl, combine the mayonnaise, mustard, prepared horseradish, Tabasco, salt, onion powder, red pepper flakes, pepper, and garlic powder. Cover, and refrigerate for at least 30 minutes to allow the flavors to develop.

2. Store any leftover mustard sauce in the refrigerator for up to 5 days.

TO MAKE THE PRETZELS
1. Proof the yeast: Put the yeast and inulin fiber in a small bowl (make sure the bowl is large enough to allow the yeast to expand). Add the warm water, and stir. Cover the bowl with a kitchen towel, and leave to rest for 10 minutes. The yeast has properly proofed when it expands and bubbles.

Continued →

2. While the yeast is proofing, line a large baking sheet with a silicone baking mat or parchment paper.

3. Put the mozzarella cheese in a large microwave-safe bowl. Microwave in 30-second increments, making sure to stir each time, until fully melted. Add the cream cheese to the melted mozzarella, and mix until combined.

4. Using a rubber spatula, stir in the coconut flour, baking powder, and xanthan gum. Add the whole eggs and proofed yeast, and combine well.

5. Once the dough comes together, lightly knead the dough with wet hands. Divide the dough into 10 equal balls, being sure to keep your hands wet so the dough doesn't stick. Roll each ball between your hands to form a pretzel stick about ¾-inch thick. Place the pretzels on the prepared baking sheet. Smooth any cracks on the surface or sides of the pretzels with your hands.

6. In a small bowl, use a whisk to beat the egg white until foamy, and brush onto the pretzels with a pastry brush. Allow the pretzels to rest and slightly rise in a warm, draft-free place for 30 minutes.

7. While the pretzels are rising, preheat the oven to 375°F.

8. Sprinkle the pretzels with coarse sea salt. Bake for 25 to 30 minutes, or until the pretzels are golden brown.

9. Allow to cool for 2 to 3 minutes in the pan, then transfer to a wire rack to cool fully.

10. Store any leftover pretzels in the refrigerator for up to 5 days, or freeze for up to 3 weeks.

Variation Tip: You can shape these into a more traditional pretzel shape if you like. Or, make these into pretzel nuggets (just pinch small pieces off the ball of dough), and serve with a keto Cheddar cheese sauce for dipping. Yum!

Per serving: Calories: 169; Total Fat: 11g; Total Carbohydrates: 8g; Net Carbs: 4g; Fiber: 4g; Protein: 10g; Erythritol: 0g
Macros: Fat: 59%; Protein: 24%; Carbs: 17%

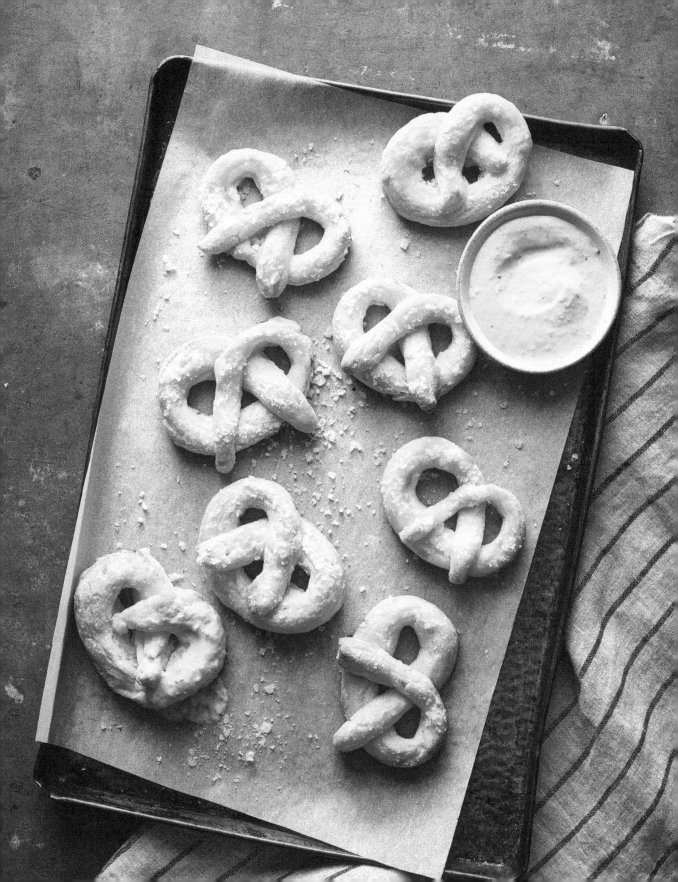

SOUTHERN SWEET CORN BREAD

MAKES 10 PIECES / PREP TIME: 10 MINUTES / COOK TIME: 30 TO 35 MINUTES, PLUS 10 MINUTES TO COOL
EQUIPMENT: 2 MIXING BOWLS, 9-INCH CAST IRON SKILLET

This Southern-style recipe is a mock corn bread, and it uses zero corn or cornmeal. Instead, by combining a corn bread flavor extract and almond meal, you can get both the flavor and texture of traditional corn bread, minus the carbs. Serve with some keto-fied fried chicken and coleslaw, and you have yourself a decadent Southern meal.

2 cups almond meal

½ cup granulated erythritol–monk fruit blend

2 teaspoons baking powder

1 teaspoon sea salt

1 cup sour cream

¼ cup heavy whipping cream

6 drops OOOFlavors corn bread extract

4 large eggs, beaten, at room temperature

½ cup (1 stick) unsalted butter, melted, plus 1 tablespoon

1. Preheat the oven to 375°F. Place the empty cast iron skillet in the preheated oven for 10 minutes.

2. In a medium bowl, combine the almond meal, erythritol–monk fruit blend, baking powder, salt, and pepper, and set aside.

3. In a large bowl, combine the sour cream, heavy whipping cream, corn bread extract, and eggs. Mix until fully combined. Add the dry ingredients to the wet ingredients, and gently stir until fully incorporated. Fold in ½ cup of melted butter, and stir gently until combined.

4. Carefully remove the hot cast iron skillet, and add the remaining 1 tablespoon of butter to it. Swirl to cover the bottom and sides. Add the corn bread batter to the hot, greased skillet. Bake for 30 to 35 minutes. Allow to cool in the pan for 10 minutes before slicing into wedges.

5. Store any leftovers in the refrigerator for up to 5 days, or freeze for 3 weeks.

Per serving: Calories: 327; Total Fat: 31g; Total Carbohydrates: 7g; Net Carbs: 5g; Fiber: 2g; Protein: 9g; Erythritol: 10g
Macros: Fat: 85%; Protein: 11%; Carbs: 4%

TEX-MEX GREEN CHILE CORN BREAD

MAKES 10 PIECES / PREP TIME: 10 MINUTES / COOK TIME: 30 TO 35 MINUTES
EQUIPMENT: 2 MIXING BOWLS, 9-INCH CAST IRON SKILLET

This mock Tex-Mex green chile corn bread is a real treat. If you're not a spice fan, replace the chiles with chopped onion and red bell peppers.

2 cups almond meal

2 tablespoons granulated erythritol–
   monk fruit blend

2 teaspoons baking powder

1 teaspoon sea salt

¼ cup heavy whipping cream

1 cup sour cream

2 (7-ounce) cans green chiles, drained
   and chopped

6 drops OOOFlavors corn bread extract

4 large eggs, beaten, at room
   temperature, at room temperature

½ cup (1 stick) unsalted butter, melted,
   plus 1 tablespoon

1 cup shredded sharp Cheddar
   cheese, divided

1. Preheat the oven to 375°F. Place the empty cast iron skillet in the preheated oven for 10 minutes.

2. In a medium bowl, combine the almond meal, erythritol–monk fruit blend, baking powder, and salt, and set aside.

3. In a large bowl, combine the heavy whipping cream, sour cream, green chiles, corn bread extract, and eggs. Mix until fully combined. Add the dry ingredients to the wet ingredients, and gently stir until fully incorporated. Fold in ½ cup of melted butter, and stir gently until combined. Then fold in ½ cup of Cheddar cheese.

4. Carefully remove the hot cast iron skillet, and add the remaining 1 tablespoon of butter to the skillet. Swirl to cover the bottom and sides. Add the corn bread batter to the hot, greased skillet. Top with the remaining ½ cup of Cheddar cheese. Bake for 30 to 35 minutes. Allow to cool in the pan for 10 minutes before slicing into wedges.

5. Store any leftovers in the refrigerator for up to 5 days, or freeze for up to 3 weeks.

Per serving: Calories: 335; Total Fat: 31g; Total Carbohydrates: 9g; Net Carbs: 6g; Fiber: 3g; Protein: 9g; Erythritol: 2g
Macros: Fat: 83%; Protein: 11%; Carbs: 6%

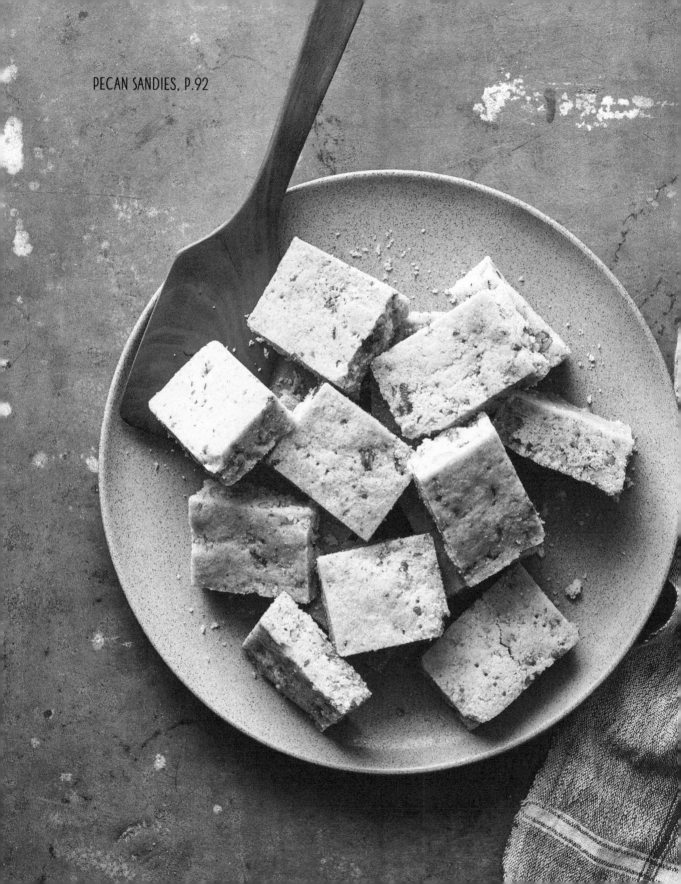

PECAN SANDIES, P.92

CHAPTER 6

COOKIES, BARS,
AND SWEET
SNACKS

PECAN SANDIES

MAKES 24 COOKIES / PREP TIME: 10 MINUTES, PLUS 45 MINUTES TO CHILL / COOK TIME: 35 TO 40 MINUTES, PLUS COOLING TIME
EQUIPMENT: 1 MIXING BOWL, 10-BY-10-INCH BAKING PAN

If you are craving a buttery, melt-in-your-mouth shortbread cookie but need it to be low in carbs, this recipe is for you. Prepare to go old-school, since this cookie dough must be made by hand to get the perfect texture. But I assure you, it's worth the extra effort.

2½ cups finely milled almond flour, measured and sifted

¾ cup granulated erythritol–monk fruit blend

½ cup finely chopped pecans (optional)

1 teaspoon baking powder

½ teaspoon sea salt

1 cup (2 sticks) unsalted butter, very cold

1½ teaspoons pure vanilla extract

1. Preheat the oven to 300°F.

2. In a medium bowl, using a whisk, combine the almond flour, erythritol–monk fruit blend, chopped pecans (if using), baking powder, and salt.

3. Take the butter out of the refrigerator, and cut it into about 30 small slices. Distribute the butter and vanilla into the flour mixture evenly. Use your fingers to rub the pieces of butter into the flour mixture, and work them into the mixture for about 5 minutes, or until the dough comes together.

4. Press the dough into a 10-by-10-inch baking pan. Place in the refrigerator to chill for at least 45 minutes.

5. Use the tines of a fork to poke holes in the top of the pecan sandies. Bake for 35 to 40 minutes, or until the edges are light golden brown.

6. Allow the shortbread to cool in the pan completely before slicing, as these cookies can be fragile.

7. Store any leftovers in the refrigerator for up to 5 days, or freeze for up to 3 weeks.

Keep in Mind: Placing the unbaked bars in the refrigerator will ensure that they have a nice crisp texture. It's important not to skip this step.

Per serving: Calories: 153; Total Fat: 15g; Total Carbohydrates: 3g; Net Carbs: 1g; Fiber: 2g; Protein: 3g; Erythritol: 6g
Macros: Fat: 88%; Protein: 8%; Carbs: 4%

LEMON COOKIES

MAKES 24 COOKIES / PREP TIME: 10 MINUTES, PLUS 30 MINUTES TO CHILL / COOK TIME: 15 MINUTES, PLUS COOLING TIME
EQUIPMENT: 3 MIXING BOWLS, ELECTRIC MIXER, LARGE BAKING SHEET

This recipe for lemon cookies creates a soft and chewy cookie bursting with tangy lemon flavor. The refreshing taste of lemon comes through boldly in this simple recipe through a combination of lemon juice, extract, and zest. It makes for the perfect spring cookie.

FOR THE COOKIES
¾ cup coconut flour

1½ teaspoons baking powder

¼ teaspoon sea salt

¾ cup granulated erythritol–monk fruit blend

8 tablespoons (1 stick) unsalted butter, at room temperature

4 ounces (about ½ cup) cream cheese, at room temperature

1 tablespoon grated lemon zest

1 teaspoon liquid lemon extract

4 large eggs, at room temperature

1 tablespoon heavy whipping cream

FOR THE LEMON ICING
½ cup confectioners' erythritol–monk fruit blend

2 tablespoons freshly squeezed lemon juice

¼ teaspoon liquid lemon extract

1 to 2 tablespoons heavy whipping cream

TO MAKE THE COOKIES

1. Preheat the oven to 350°F. Line a large baking sheet with a silicone baking mat or parchment paper.

2. In a medium bowl, mix together the coconut flour, baking powder, and salt.

3. In a large bowl, using an electric mixer on medium speed, cream the erythritol–monk fruit blend, butter, cream cheese, lemon zest, and lemon extract. Add the eggs one at a time, beating well after each addition. Add the heavy whipping cream, and mix until fully incorporated. Add the dry ingredients to the wet batter, and mix well until the dough is formed.

4. Chill the dough for 30 minutes in the refrigerator before baking.

Continued →

5. Using a tablespoon or a small cookie scoop, measure out the cookie dough. Roll each scoop of cookie dough into a small ball. Lay the balls out evenly on the baking sheet. Lightly flatten the balls with your palms. Bake for 15 minutes, or until lightly browned around the edges.

6. Allow to cool completely on a wire rack before icing.

TO MAKE THE LEMON ICING AND FINISH THE COOKIES

1. In a medium bowl, combine the confectioners' erythritol–monk fruit blend with the lemon juice and lemon extract. Add 1 tablespoon heavy whipping cream to thin the icing, and add another tablespoon if necessary.

2. Drizzle over tops of the fully cooled cookies, and allow the icing to set for about 15 minutes before eating.

3. Store any leftovers in the refrigerator for up to 5 days, or freeze for up to 3 weeks.

Variation Tip: For a different flavor, you can make these into almond cookies. For the cookies, simply replace the lemon extract with almond extract, and remove the lemon zest. For the icing, remove the lemon juice, increase the heavy whipping cream to 3 tablespoons, and replace the lemon extract with almond extract. After icing the cookies, you can sprinkle 2 tablespoons of slivered almonds on top before the icing sets.

Per serving: Calories: 82; Total Fat: 7g; Total Carbohydrates: 3g; Net Carbs: 1g; Fiber: 2g; Protein: 2g; Erythritol: 9g
Macros: Fat: 77%; Protein: 10%; Carbs: 13%

CHOCOLATE CHUNK COOKIES

MAKES 16 COOKIES / PREP TIME: 10 MINUTES / COOK TIME: 10 TO 15 MINUTES, PLUS COOLING TIME
EQUIPMENT: 1 MIXING BOWL, ELECTRIC MIXER, LARGE BAKING SHEET

The chunks of sugar-free chocolate make this a bold cookie. These buttery cookies have a chewy texture that is achieved by using a little unflavored gelatin in the batter.

12 tablespoons (1½ sticks) unsalted butter, at room temperature

½ cup golden or brown granulated erythritol–monk fruit blend

½ cup granulated erythritol–monk fruit blend

1 tablespoon sugar-free maple syrup

½ teaspoon pure vanilla extract

2 large eggs, at room tempaterature

1 tablespoon unflavored gelatin powder

2 cups finely milled almond flour, measured and sifted

¼ cup coconut flour

2 teaspoons baking powder

¼ teaspoon salt

½ cup roughly chopped sugar-free chocolate bar

1. Preheat the oven to 350°F. Line a large baking sheet with a silicone baking mat or parchment paper.

2. In a large bowl, using an electric mixer on medium speed, beat the butter, golden erythritol–monk fruit blend erythritol–monk fruit blend, maple syrup, and vanilla until light and fluffy. Add the eggs one at a time, mixing well after each addition. Sprinkle in the gelatin powder, and combine well.

3. Mix in the almond flour, coconut flour, baking powder, and salt. Fold in the chocolate chunks.

4. Drop the dough onto the baking sheet by heaping tablespoons spaced about 2 inches apart. Flatten the cookies slightly with your palm.

5. Bake for 12 to 15 minutes, or until golden. Allow to cool completely on a wire rack before eating or storing.

6. Store any leftovers in the refrigerator for up to 5 days, or freeze for up to 3 weeks.

Variation Tip: Make these orange–chocolate chunk cookies by replacing the vanilla extract with orange extract.

Per serving: Calories: 211; Total Fat: 19g; Total Carbohydrates: 9g; Net Carbs: 6g; Fiber: 3g; Protein: 5g; Erythritol: 12g
Macros: Fat: 81%; Protein: 9%; Carbs: 10%

PEANUT BUTTER–CHOCOLATE CHIP COOKIES

MAKES 16 COOKIES / PREP TIME: 10 MINUTES / COOK TIME: 10 TO 15 MINUTES, PLUS 15 MINUTES TO COOL
EQUIPMENT: 1 MIXING BOWL, ELECTRIC MIXER, LARGE BAKING SHEET

These cookies are packed with peanut butter and chocolate and offer the best of both worlds. I've always loved this combo! This low-carb cookie recipe pairs these flavors well for a tasty keto-friendly treat.

1 cup sugar-free all-natural peanut butter

1 cup granulated erythritol–monk fruit blend

8 tablespoons (1 stick) unsalted butter, softened

1 large egg, at room temperature

1 cup finely milled almond flour, measured and sifted

1 teaspoon baking powder

½ teaspoon sea salt

½ cup sugar-free chocolate chips

Sea salt flakes (optional)

1. Preheat the oven to 350°F. Line a large baking sheet with a silicone baking mat or parchment paper.

2. In a large bowl, using an electric mixer, beat the peanut butter, erythritol–monk fruit blend, butter, and egg until well combined. Add the almond flour, baking powder, and salt. Beat the mixture until fully incorporated. Fold in the chocolate chips.

3. Using a tablespoon or small cookie scoop, evenly space spoonfuls of the cookie dough on the prepared baking sheet. Lightly flatten the cookies with the back of the spoon, then use the tines of a fork to make a crisscross design. Sprinkle with sea salt flakes (if using).

4. Bake for 10 to 12 minutes, or until lightly browned around the edges.

5. Allow to cool completely on the baking sheet for at least 15 minutes before eating and storing, as these cookies can be fragile.

6. Store any leftovers in the refrigerator for up to 5 days, or freeze for up to 3 weeks.

Per serving: Calories: 225; Total Fat: 20g; Total Carbohydrates: 9g; Net Carbs: 7g; Fiber: 2g; Protein: 6g; Erythritol: 12g
Macros: Fat: 80%; Protein: 11%; Carbs: 9%

DOUBLE CHOCOLATE PEPPERMINT COOKIES

MAKES 16 COOKIES / PREP TIME: 15 MINUTES / COOK TIME: 15 TO 20 MINUTES, PLUS COOLING TIME
EQUIPMENT: 3 MIXING BOWLS, ELECTRIC MIXER, LARGE BAKING SHEET

Am I the only one who associates the classic flavor of chocolate and peppermint with the winter holidays? These festive, double chocolate, soft-baked cookies remind me of thin mints. They get their infusion of mint flavor from peppermint extract in the batter and a sprinkling of crushed sugar-free peppermint starlight mints on top of the chocolate icing. The addition of the espresso in this recipe really deepens the flavor and brings out the chocolate. These cookies will be a great addition to your holiday cookie tray.

FOR THE COOKIES

2 ounces (2 squares) unsweetened baking chocolate
8 ounces (about 1 cup) cream cheese, at room temperature
1 cup granulated erythritol–monk fruit blend
8 tablespoons (1 stick) unsalted butter, at room temperature
1 teaspoon liquid peppermint extract
4 large eggs, at room temperature
1 cup coconut flour
¼ cup unsweetened cocoa powder
2 teaspoons baking powder
1 teaspoon instant espresso coffee
¼ teaspoon sea salt

FOR THE ICING AND TOPPING

4 tablespoons (½ stick) unsalted butter
2 ounces (2 squares) unsweetened baking chocolate
½ cup confectioners' erythritol–monk fruit blend
1 teaspoon coconut oil
1 teaspoon instant espresso coffee
Pinch sea salt
5 sugar-free peppermint candies, crushed

TO MAKE THE COOKIES

1. Preheat the oven to 350°F. Line a large baking sheet with a silicone baking mat or parchment paper.

2. Put the baking chocolate in a microwave-safe bowl. Microwave in 10-second increments, making sure to stir each time, until fully melted.

Continued →

3. In a large bowl, using an electric mixer on high speed, combine the cream cheese, erythritol–monk fruit blend, butter, and peppermint extract. Add the eggs one at a time, making sure they are fully incorporated into the batter. Add the chocolate, and beat the dough until it's very well mixed. Mix in the coconut flour, unsweetened cocoa powder, baking powder, instant espresso coffee, and salt.

4. Using a tablespoon or small cookie scoop, evenly space spoonfuls of the cookie dough on the prepared baking sheet. Slightly flatten the cookies using your palms. Bake for 15 to 20 minutes, being careful not to overbake. Place the cookies on a wire rack to cool completely before icing.

TO MAKE THE ICING AND TOPPING AND DECORATE THE COOKIES

1. Put the butter and baking chocolate in a microwave-safe bowl. Microwave in 10-second increments, making sure to stir each time, until fully melted. Add the confectioners' erythritol–monk fruit blend and stir. Mix in the coconut oil, instant espresso coffee, and salt.

2. Once the cookies have cooled completely, spread about 1 teaspoon of icing on the top of each cookie. Sprinkle the top of each cookie with the peppermint candies. Make sure to add the candies before the icing sets so that they stick to the cookies.

3. Allow to set for at least 5 minutes before eating.

4. Store any leftovers in the refrigerator for up to 5 days, or freeze for up to 3 weeks.

Keep in Mind: You can also use a double boiler or a glass mixing bowl set on top of a medium saucepan with simmering water to melt the chocolate if you'd rather not use the microwave.

Per serving: Calories: 220; Total Fat: 20g; Total Carbohydrates: 10g; Net Carbs: 5g; Fiber: 5g; Protein: 5g; Erythritol: 17g
Macros: Fat: 82%; Protein: 9%; Carbs: 9%

CHOCOLATE CHIP BROWNIES

MAKES 16 BROWNIES / PREP TIME: 10 MINUTES / COOK TIME: 20 TO 25 MINUTES, PLUS 30 MINUTES TO COOL
EQUIPMENT: 2 MIXING BOWLS, MEDIUM SAUCEPAN, 8-BY-8-INCH BAKING PAN

When chocolate cravings are running high, these chocolate chip brownies are here to come to your rescue. Not only are these keto-friendly brownies flat-out delicious, but also they are a breeze to make. The teaspoon of instant coffee isn't strictly necessary, but it does enhance the chocolaty flavor of the brownies—you won't be sorry you tried it!

10 tablespoons unsalted butter, plus more to grease the pan

1¼ cups granulated erythritol–monk fruit blend

¾ cup dark unsweetened cocoa powder

1 ounce (1 square) unsweetened baking chocolate, roughly chopped

1 teaspoon instant coffee (optional)

¼ teaspoon sea salt

3 large eggs, at room temperature

2 teaspoons pure vanilla extract

¾ cup almond flour, measured and sifted

1 teaspoon baking powder

½ cup sugar-free chocolate chips

1. Preheat the oven to 325°F. Lightly grease the 8-by-8-inch baking pan with butter.

2. In a medium saucepan, bring 1 cup water to a boil over medium-high heat. Set a glass mixing bowl over the saucepan, making sure the bowl doesn't touch the water. Add to the bowl the butter, erythritol–monk fruit blend, unsweetened cocoa powder, unsweetened baking chocolate, instant coffee (if using), and salt to the bowl. Whisk occasionally until fully melted and combined. Allow the mixture to cool slightly, and pour it into a large mixing bowl.

3. Add the eggs one at a time to the chocolate mixture. Add the vanilla, and mix well. Add the almond flour and baking powder, and gently stir with a rubber spatula until just combined. Fold in the chocolate chips.

Continued →

4. Pour the brownie mixture into the prepared pan, and bake for 20 to 25 minutes.

5. Allow the brownies to cool for at least 30 minutes in the pan before slicing.

6. Store any leftovers in the refrigerator for up to 5 days, or freeze for up to 3 weeks.

Keep in Mind: It's important not to overbake your brownies. The brownies should be set in the middle but still jiggle a bit when the pan is moved. They'll set more as they cool.

Per serving: Calories: 160; Total Fat: 14g; Total Carbohydrates: 9g; Net Carbs: 6g; Fiber: 3g; Protein: 3g; Erythritol: 15g
Macros: Fat: 79%; Protein: 8%; Carbs: 13%

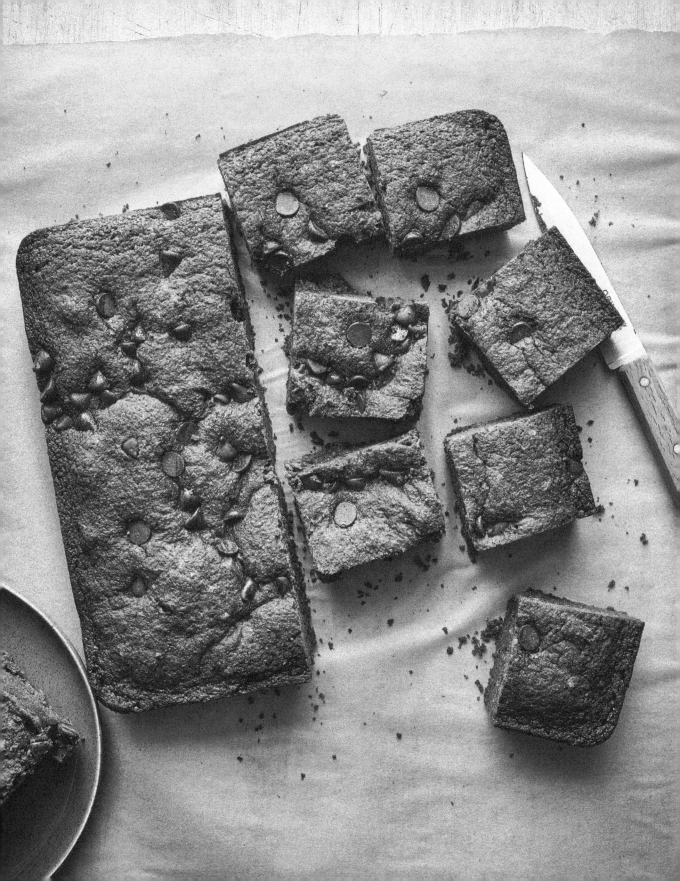

SNICKERDOODLE BARS

MAKES 24 BARS / PREP TIME: 10 MINUTES / COOK TIME: 30 TO 40 MINUTES, PLUS COOLING TIME
EQUIPMENT: 2 MIXING BOWLS, ELECTRIC MIXER, 10-BY-10-INCH BAKING PAN

These snickerdoodle bars are buttery, soft, and chewy, with the perfect amount of tang, which is a sign of a good snickerdoodle. Using xanthan gum is optional, but it does give these bars their chewy texture.

8 tablespoons (1 stick) unsalted butter, at room temperature, plus more to grease the pan

2 cups granulated erythritol–monk fruit blend, plus 3 tablespoons

8 ounces (about 1 cup) cream cheese, at room temperature

2 teaspoons pure vanilla extract

5 large eggs, at room temperature

1 cup finely milled almond flour, measured and sifted

⅓ cup coconut flour

½ teaspoon baking soda

½ teaspoon cream of tartar

½ teaspoon xanthan gum (optional)

¼ teaspoon sea salt

2 teaspoons ground cinnamon

1. Preheat the oven to 350°F. Grease a 10-by-10-inch baking pan with butter.

2. In a large bowl, using an electric mixer on medium speed, beat 2 cups of erythritol–monk fruit blend, the cream cheese, butter, and vanilla. Add the eggs one at a time, mixing well after each addition. Fold in the almond flour, coconut flour, baking soda, cream of tartar, xanthan gum (if using) and salt.

3. Pour the batter into the prepared pan, and spread evenly.

4. In a small bowl, combine the remaining 3 tablespoons of erythritol–monk fruit blend and the cinnamon. Sprinkle the mixture on top of the batter. Bake for 30 to 35 minutes, or until golden brown.

5. Allow to cool completely in the pan on a wire rack before slicing into bars.

6. Store any leftovers in the refrigerator for up to 5 days, or freeze for up to 3 weeks.

Keep in Mind: Cream of tartar is an essential ingredient because it gives these snickerdoodle bars their classic tangy flavor and is also used as a rising agent.

Per serving: Calories: 116; Total Fat: 11g; Total Carbohydrates: 3g; Net Carbs: 2g; Fiber: 1g; Protein: 3g; Erythritol: 18g
Macros: Fat: 85%; Protein: 10%; Carbs: 5%

CINNAMON ROLLS WITH CREAM CHEESE ICING

MAKES 9 ROLLS / PREP TIME: 20 MINUTES, PLUS RISING TIME / COOK TIME: 15 TO 25 MINUTES
EQUIPMENT: 5 MIXING BOWLS, COFFEE GRINDER, 9-BY-9-INCH BAKING PAN, LARGE BAKING SHEET

In my opinion, there is nothing like the smell of homemade cinnamon rolls baking in the oven. These cinnamon rolls are as close to their high-carb counterparts as you can get without the aid of gluten. The dough uses a combination of almond and coconut flours, flax meal, psyllium husk powder, and yeast for one delicious keto-friendly treat.

FOR THE CINNAMON ROLLS

1 tablespoon yeast

1 tablespoon inulin fiber or sugar

⅛ teaspoon ground ginger

3 tablespoons warm water, plus ¾ cup

¼ cup golden flax meal

2 large eggs, at room temperature

¼ cup coconut flour

1½ tablespoons unsalted butter, melted

1¼ cups finely milled almond flour, measured and sifted

¼ cup psyllium husk powder

2 teaspoons baking powder

¼ cup granulated erythritol–monk fruit blend

2 tablespoons ground cinnamon

2 tablespoons salted butter, softened, plus more to grease the pan

FOR THE CREAM CHEESE ICING

¼ cup cream cheese, at room temperature

¼ cup confectioners' erythritol–monk fruit blend

3 tablespoons unsalted butter, at room temperature

1 teaspoon pure vanilla extract

¼ teaspoon sea salt

2 to 3 tablespoons heavy whipping cream

Continued →

TO MAKE THE CINNAMON ROLLS

1. Proof the yeast: Put the yeast, inulin fiber, and ginger in a small bowl (make sure the bowl is large enough to allow the yeast to expand). Add 3 tablespoons of warm water, and stir. Cover the bowl with a kitchen towel, and leave to rest for 10 minutes. The yeast has properly proofed when it expands and bubbles.

2. While the yeast is proofing, grind the flax meal in a coffee grinder until it's a fine powder. Set aside.

3. In a medium bowl, whisk together the eggs, coconut flour, and melted butter. Using a rubber spatula, add the proofed yeast, and combine well. Set aside.

4. In a large bowl, sift together the almond flour, flax meal powder, psyllium husk powder, and baking powder. Add the remaining ¾ cup of warm water and the yeast–coconut flour mixture to the dry ingredients. Combine well to form a dough. Cover the bowl with a kitchen towel, and let rest for 10 minutes.

5. To make the filling, in a small bowl, combine the granulated erythritol–monk fruit blend and cinnamon.

6. With wet hands, spread the dough into a 7-by 9-inch rectangle on a sheet of parchment paper. Using a pastry brush, spread the softened salted butter on the dough and then sprinkle the filling on top of the butter. Be sure to leave half an inch along the top free of filling to help when rolling the dough.

7. Starting from the long end, roll the dough as tightly as you can using the parchment paper to help. Pinch the end closed all along the roll, using wet fingers. Using a wet, sharp knife, cut the dough into 9 even pieces.

8. Grease a 9-by-9-inch baking pan with butter. Add the rolls to the baking pan, cut-side up, and press them down softly with your palms. Cover with a kitchen towel, and allow to rise in a draft-free area for 50 minutes to 1 hour or until they have almost doubled in size. The time will depend on many factors based on where you are located, so continue to check on them every so often.

9. While the dough is rising, preheat the oven to 400°F.

10. Once the rolls have expanded, place the baking pan on a large baking sheet, and bake for 15 to 25 minutes, or until the rolls are golden. If the tops start to brown too quickly, cover loosely with aluminum foil until the rolls are cooked through.

TO MAKE THE CREAM CHEESE ICING AND FINISH THE ROLLS

1. Cream the cream cheese, confectioners' erythritol–monk fruit blend, and butter. While mixing, add the vanilla and salt. Then gradually add 2 tablespoons heavy whipping cream. If the icing is too thick, add more heavy whipping cream 1 teaspoon at a time.

2. Use a spatula to spread the icing on top immediately after removing the rolls from the oven, and only to the ones you plan to eat that day.

3. Store any leftovers, without icing, in an airtight container for up to 4 days in the refrigerator. After reheating, add the icing on top while still warm.

Variation Tip: You can use this dough to make cinnamon roll bites, which will save a lot of time. Form 1½-inch balls from the dough, and dip each ball in melted butter, then toss in the cinnamon mix. Place the balls into a 9-inch cake pan, cover with a kitchen towel, and allow to rise for 50 minutes to 1 hour. Bake at 400°F until golden brown, or 15 to 25 minutes. Thin the cream cheese icing with a bit more cream, and use it as a dipping sauce for the cinnamon roll bites.

Per serving: Calories: 268; Total Fat: 22g; Total Carbohydrates: 13g; Net Carbs: 4g; Fiber: 9g; Protein: 7g; Erythritol: 9g
Macros: Fat: 74%; Protein: 10%; Carbs: 16%

HAZELNUT-CHOCOLATE SNACK CAKES

MAKES 24 CAKES / PREP TIME: 10 MINUTES / COOK TIME: 30 TO 35 MINUTES, PLUS COOLING TIME
EQUIPMENT: 1 MIXING BOWL, ELECTRIC MIXER, 9-BY-13-INCH BAKING PAN

These lovely snack cakes combine hazelnut flour, unsweetened cocoa powder, and sugar-free chocolate chips for one delicious dessert. If you're a fan of chocolate hazelnut spread, then you're in for a treat with this cake. Enjoy the flavor combination of pure decadence without the fuss or worry of carbs. This easy chocolate hazelnut snack cake is perfect to add to a lunch box for a sweet treat or to serve in the afternoon with coffee and tea.

2 cups granulated erythritol–monk fruit blend

8 ounces (about 1 cup) cream cheese, at room temperature

8 tablespoons (1 stick) unsalted butter, at room temperature, plus more to grease the pan

1 teaspoon liquid hazelnut extract

5 large eggs, at room temperature

1 cup hazelnut flour

⅓ cup coconut flour

¼ cup unsweetened cocoa powder

1½ teaspoons baking powder

¼ teaspoon sea salt

1 cup chopped hazelnuts

½ cup sugar-free chocolate chips

½ cup roughly chopped unsweetened baking chocolate

1. Preheat the oven to 350°F. Grease a 9-by-13-inch baking pan with butter.

2. In a large bowl, using an electric mixer, beat the erythritol–monk fruit blend, cream cheese, butter, and hazelnut extract. Add the eggs one at a time, and mix well after each addition to make sure the eggs are well incorporated into the batter. Fold in the hazelnut flour, coconut flour, unsweetened cocoa powder, baking powder, and salt. Using a spatula, stir in the hazelnuts, chocolate chips, and unsweetened baking chocolate.

3. Pour the batter into the prepared pan, and bake for 30 to 35 minutes, or until golden brown.

4. Allow the cake to cool completely in the pan, then cut into 24 individual snack cakes.

5. Store any leftovers in the refrigerator for up to 5 days, or freeze for up to 3 weeks.

Variation Tip: Instead of adding the sugar-free chocolate chips and hazelnuts, you can make a simple hazelnut glaze. Combine ½ cup confectioners' erythritol–monk fruit blend, 2 to 3 tablespoons heavy whipping cream, and ¼ teaspoon hazelnut extract. Start with 2 tablespoons heavy whipping cream, and add additional tablespoons if the glaze is too thick. Drizzle the glaze over the completely cooled snack cakes.

Per serving: Calories: 187; Total Fat: 17g; Total Carbohydrates: 8g; Net Carbs: 5g; Fiber: 3g; Protein: 4g; Erythritol: 16g
Macros: Fat: 82%; Protein: 9%; Carbs: 9%

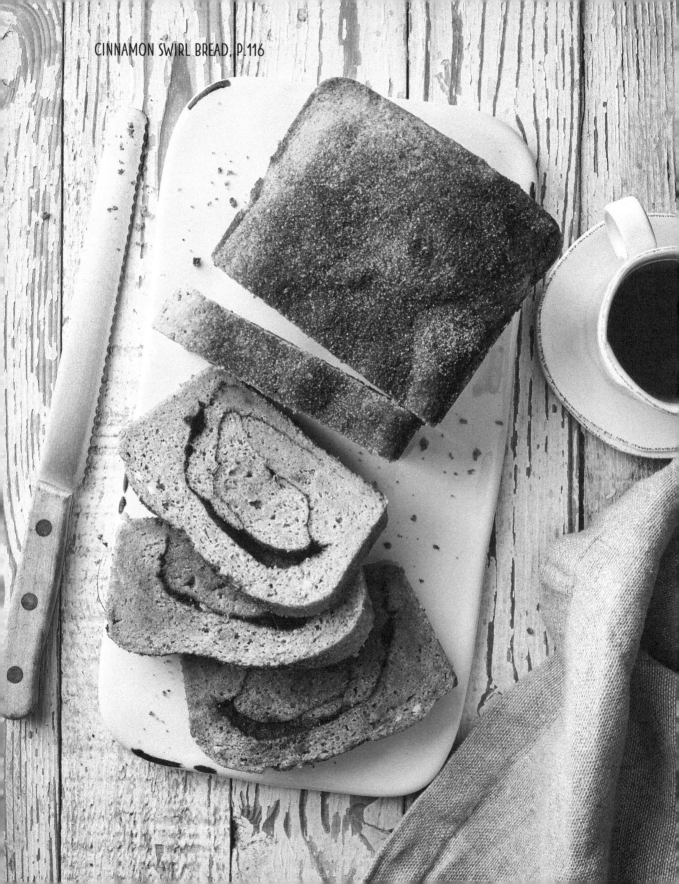

CINNAMON SWIRL BREAD, P. 116

CHAPTER 7

ʃʅʅ

SWEET LOAVES
AND DESSERT CAKES

DAIRY-FREE ZUCCHINI BREAD WITH VANILLA ICING

MAKES 10 SLICES / PREP TIME: 10 MINUTES / COOK TIME: 25 TO 35 MINUTES, PLUS COOLING TIME
EQUIPMENT: 3 MIXING BOWLS, ELECTRIC MIXER, 9-BY-5-INCH LOAF PAN

Tender, moist, and low in carbs, this healthy zucchini bread will help you make use of a bountiful zucchini harvest. The fact that it uses zero dairy means more people can enjoy this classic treat. What makes this recipe stand out from its high-carb counterparts is that it's not loaded with sugar and manufactured oil. It's both flavorful and good for you!

FOR THE BREAD
½ cup coconut oil, solid
½ cup granulated erythritol–monk fruit blend
¼ cup brown or golden granulated erythritol–monk fruit blend
2 large eggs, at room temperature
¼ cup coconut milk or almond milk
½ teaspoon pure vanilla extract
¾ cup grated zucchini, lightly blotted with a paper towel
1½ cups finely milled almond flour, measured and sifted
1¼ teaspoons baking powder
1 teaspoon ground cinnamon
¼ teaspoon ground nutmeg
¼ teaspoon sea salt
¾ cup chopped walnuts

FOR THE VANILLA ICING
½ cup confectioners' erythritol–monk fruit blend
2 to 3 tablespoons coconut milk or almond milk
¼ teaspoon pure vanilla extract

TO MAKE THE BREAD

1. Preheat the oven to 350°F. Line a 9-by-5-inch loaf pan with parchment paper.

2. In a large bowl, using an electric mixer, cream the coconut oil, erythritol–monk fruit blend, and brown erythritol–monk fruit blend until light and fluffy. Beat in the eggs one at a time. Add the coconut milk and vanilla, and combine well. Add the zucchini, and mix well until fully combined.

3. In a medium bowl, combine the almond flour, baking powder, cinnamon, nutmeg, and salt.

4. Add the dry ingredients to the wet ingredients, and combine until well mixed. Fold in the walnuts.

5. Pour the batter into the prepared loaf pan. Bake for 25 to 35 minutes, or until a toothpick inserted into the center comes out clean.

6. Allow the loaf to cool in the pan for 10 minutes and then transfer to a wire rack to cool fully before icing.

7. Store leftovers in the refrigerator for up to 5 days or freeze for up to 3 weeks.

TO MAKE THE VANILLA ICING AND FINISH THE BREAD

1. In a small bowl, combine the confectioners' erythritol–monk fruit blend, coconut milk, and vanilla.

2. Once the bread has fully cooled, drizzle the icing on top.

3. Store any leftovers in the refrigerator for up to 5 days, or freeze for up to 3 weeks.

Ingredient Tip: Do not peel the zucchini before grating. To properly grate it, use the large holes of the box grater, then simply blot the extra moisture with a paper towel. Make sure to lightly pack when measuring.

Per serving: Calories: 271; Total Fat: 27g; Total Carbohydrates: 6g; Net Carbs: 3g; Fiber: 3g; Protein: 7g; Erythritol: 22g
Macros: Fat: 89%; Protein: 10%; Carbs: 1%

ICED CRANBERRY-GINGERBREAD LOAF

MAKES 10 SLICES / PREP TIME: 10 MINUTES / COOK TIME: 45 MINUTES TO 1 HOUR, PLUS COOLING TIME
EQUIPMENT: 3 MIXING BOWLS, ELECTRIC MIXER, 9-BY-5-INCH LOAF PAN

The winter holidays can be especially challenging for anyone doing a keto diet, but with the help of this Iced Cranberry-Gingerbread Loaf, you can enjoy a seasonal treat without having to worry about being kicked out of ketosis. Toast this lovely loaf, and enjoy a slice with your favorite hot beverage for a guilt-free indulgence.

FOR THE LOAF

1¼ cups finely milled almond flour, measured and sifted
1½ teaspoons baking powder
¼ teaspoon sea salt
1 tablespoon ground ginger
2 teaspoons ground cinnamon
½ teaspoon ground nutmeg
¼ teaspoon ground cloves
¼ teaspoon ground allspice
⅛ teaspoon pepper
4 ounces (about ½ cup) cream cheese, at room temperature
½ cup brown or golden granulated erythritol–monk fruit blend
4 tablespoons (½ stick) unsalted butter, at room temperature
1 teaspoon pure vanilla extract
4 large eggs, at room temperature
1 cup whole cranberries, fresh or frozen
¼ cup chopped walnuts

FOR THE CREAM CHEESE ICING

4 ounces (about ½ cup) cream cheese, at room temperature
2 tablespoons unsalted butter, at room temperature
½ confectioners' erythritol–monk fruit blend
¼ teaspoon pure vanilla extract
Pinch salt
½ cup heavy whipping cream

TO MAKE THE LOAF

1. Preheat the oven to 350°F. Line a 9-by-5-inch loaf pan with parchment paper.

2. In a medium bowl, combine the almond flour, baking powder, salt, ginger, cinnamon, nutmeg, cloves, allspice, and pepper. Set aside.

3. In a large bowl, using an electric mixer, mix together the cream cheese, erythritol–monk fruit blend, butter, and vanilla until the mixture is light and fluffy. Add the eggs one at a time, mixing after each addition and making sure to scrape the bowl down with a rubber spatula several times.

4. Add the dry ingredients to the wet ingredients, and combine until well incorporated. Fold in the cranberries.

5. Spread the batter into the prepared loaf pan, and sprinkle the top with the walnuts. Bake for 45 minutes to 1 hour, or until a toothpick inserted into the center comes out clean.

6. Allow the loaf to cool for about 10 minutes before taking it out of the pan. Allow to cool completely before icing.

TO MAKE THE CREAM CHEESE ICING AND FINISH THE LOAF

1. In a large bowl, using an electric mixer, beat the cream cheese, butter, and vanilla until light and fluffy. Add the confectioners' erythritol–monk fruit blend and salt, and mix gently until just combined.

2. Add the heavy whipping cream a couple of tablespoons at a time, and beat until fully combined.

3. Once the loaf has fully cooled, spread the icing on top, and serve.

4. Store any leftovers in the refrigerator for up to 5 days, or freeze for up to 3 weeks.

Ingredient Tip: If you can't find cranberries, because they aren't in season or are hard to come by in your area, you can leave them out and still enjoy a delicious gingerbread loaf all year round.

Per serving: Calories: 317; Total Fat: 30g; Total Carbohydrates: 7g; Net Carbs: 5g; Fiber: 2g; Protein: 8g; Erythritol: 17g
Macros: Fat: 85%; Protein: 10%; Carbs: 5%

PUMPKIN SPICE LOAF WITH MAPLE ICING

MAKES 10 SLICES / PREP TIME: 10 MINUTES / COOK TIME: 45 TO 50 MINUTES, PLUS COOLING TIME
EQUIPMENT: 3 MIXING BOWLS, ELECTRIC MIXER, 9-BY-5-INCH LOAF PAN

When coffee houses start sharing their pumpkin spice goodies, you won't feel like your willpower has zero chance of winning, because this simple yet tasty recipe will make sure you don't succumb to the seasonal temptation. Enjoy this flavorful loaf all pumpkin season long, and reap the rewards of staying on the keto plan. This recipe doubles well, making it great for holiday parties and meal planning.

FOR THE LOAF
8 tablespoons (1 stick) unsalted butter, at room temperature, plus more to grease the pan

1½ cups finely milled almond flour, measured and sifted

1½ tablespoons ground cinnamon

1½ tablespoons ground ginger

1½ teaspoons pumpkin pie spice

1½ teaspoons baking powder

¼ teaspoon ground nutmeg

¼ teaspoon sea salt

⅛ teaspoon ground cloves

¾ cup granulated erythritol–monk fruit blend

4 ounces (about ½ cup) cream cheese, at room temperature

¼ cup brown or golden granulated erythritol–monk fruit blend

1 teaspoon pure vanilla extract

½ cup canned pumpkin purée

3 large eggs, at room temperature

FOR THE MAPLE ICING
½ cup confectioners' erythritol–monk fruit blend

1 teaspoon ground cinnamon

¼ cup heavy whipping cream

1 tablespoon sugar-free maple syrup

TO MAKE THE LOAF

1. Preheat the oven to 350°F. Generously grease a 9-by-5-inch loaf pan with butter.

2. In a medium bowl, sift together the almond flour, cinnamon, ginger, pumpkin pie spice, baking powder, nutmeg, salt, and cloves. Set aside.

3. In a large bowl, using an electric mixer on high speed, beat the erythritol–monk fruit blend, butter, cream cheese, brown erythritol–monk fruit blend, and vanilla. Beat for 2 to 3 minutes, or until light and creamy. Add the pumpkin purée, and mix until just incorporated.

4. Alternate adding the eggs one at a time with the dry ingredients. Be sure to mix thoroughly after each addition. Scrape down the sides of the bowl periodically.

5. Pour the batter into the prepared pan, and bake for 45 to 50 minutes, or until a toothpick inserted into the center comes out clean.

6. Allow to cool in the pan for 10 minutes before removing. Allow to cool completely before icing.

TO MAKE THE MAPLE ICING AND FINISH THE LOAF

1. In a medium bowl, combine the confectioners' erythritol–monk fruit blend and cinnamon.

2. Whisk in the heavy whipping cream, making sure to fully incorporate the mixture. Add the maple syrup, and mix well.

3. Once the loaf has fully cooled, spread the icing on top, and serve.

4. Store any leftovers in an airtight container in the refrigerator for up to 7 days, or freeze for up to 30 days.

Ingredient Tip: You can easily make your own pumpkin pie spice at home. Mix together 4 teaspoons ground cinnamon, 2 teaspoons ground ginger, 1 teaspoon ground cloves, 1 teaspoon ground allspice, and ½ teaspoon ground nutmeg. Store in an airtight container in a cool, dry place for up to 6 months.

Per serving: Calories: 270; Total Fat: 25g; Total Carbohydrates: 7g; Net Carbs: 4g; Fiber: 3g; Protein: 7g; Erythritol: 26g
Macros: Fat: 83%; Protein: 10%; Carbs: 7%

CINNAMON SWIRL BREAD

MAKES 12 SLICES / PREP TIME: 10 MINUTES / COOK TIME: 45 MINUTES TO 1 HOUR, PLUS 30 TO 40 MINUTES TO COOL
EQUIPMENT: 2 MIXING BOWLS, ELECTRIC MIXER, 9-BY-5-INCH LOAF PAN

Ah, the smell of homemade cinnamon swirl bread being baked is unmatched. However, traditional cinnamon bread is loaded with tons of carbs and has no place in a ketogenic lifestyle. Thankfully, you can enjoy this classic flavor without the worry of carbs ruining your hard work with this easy, delicious keto recipe.

8 tablespoons (1 stick) unsalted butter, melted and cooled, plus more to grease the pan

1 cup coconut milk

6 large eggs, at room tempaterature

1 cup finely milled almond flour, measured and sifted

¾ cup granulated erythritol–monk fruit blend, divided

½ cup coconut flour

½ cup psyllium husk powder

1½ teaspoons baking powder

½ teaspoon sea salt

2 tablespoons ground cinnamon

1. Preheat the oven to 350°F. Grease a 9-by-5-inch loaf pan with butter.

2. In a large bowl, using an electric mixer, combine the coconut milk and butter, then add the eggs one at a time. Add the almond flour, ½ cup of erythritol–monk fruit blend, the coconut flour, psyllium husk powder, baking powder, and salt. Mix the batter on medium speed for about 2 minutes, or until fully incorporated. This batter will be thick.

3. In a small bowl, combine the remaining ¼ cup of erythritol–monk fruit blend and the cinnamon.

4. Place half the batter into the loaf pan. Sprinkle the cinnamon mixture on top, reserving 2 teaspoons. Add the other half of the batter. Sprinkle the top of the bread with the reserved cinnamon mixture. Bake for 45 minutes to 1 hour, or until a toothpick inserted into the center comes out clean.

5. Allow to cool for about 10 minutes before removing from the pan. Place on a wire rack for another 20 to 30 minutes to fully cool before slicing.

6. Store any leftovers in the refrigerator for up to 5 days, or freeze for up to 3 weeks.

Variation Tip: You can make a vanilla icing to drizzle on the top of this cinnamon swirl bread by combining ½ cup confectioners' erythritol–monk fruit blend with 2 to 3 tablespoons heavy whipping cream and ¼ teaspoon pure vanilla extract. Ice the loaf after it is completely cool so the icing doesn't melt.

Per serving: Calories: 210; Total Fat: 16g; Total Carbohydrates: 13g; Net Carbs: 5g; Fiber: 8g; Protein: 6g; Erythritol: 12g
Macros: Fat: 69%; Protein: 11%; Carbs: 20%

CHOCOLATE CHIP BANANA BREAD

MAKES 12 SLICES / PREP TIME: 5 TO 10 MINUTES / COOK TIME: 35 TO 40 MINUTES, PLUS COOLING TIME
EQUIPMENT: 2 MIXING BOWLS, COFFEE GRINDER, ELECTRIC MIXER, 9-BY-5-INCH LOAF PAN

Before you tell me that bananas are not keto, let me make it clear that no real bananas were used to make this delicious loaf. What's my secret? It's a matter of getting the perfect texture and boosting the flavor with a legit banana flavor concentrate. The addition of sugar-free chocolate chips takes this banana bread to the next level. Serve this as a snack at your next gathering—I promise no one will be able to tell the difference!

½ cup golden flax meal

1 cup finely milled almond flour, measured and sifted

½ cup coconut flour

1 tablespoon baking powder

1 tablespoon psyllium husk powder

2 teaspoons ground cinnamon

¼ teaspoon ground nutmeg

¼ teaspoon sea salt

¾ cup brown or golden granulated erythritol–monk fruit blend

½ cup coconut oil, melted

2 tablespoons sugar-free maple syrup

5 or 6 drops liquid banana extract

1 teaspoon pure vanilla extract

4 large eggs, at room tempaterature

½ cup coconut or almond milk

½ cup sugar-free chocolate chips, divided

1. Preheat the oven to 350°F. Line a 9-by-5-inch loaf pan with parchment paper.

2. In a coffee grinder, grind the flax meal until it's a fine powder.

3. In a medium bowl, combine the flax meal powder, almond flour, coconut flour, baking powder, psyllium husk powder, cinnamon, nutmeg, and salt. Set aside.

4. In a large bowl, combine the erythritol–monk fruit blend, coconut oil, maple syrup, banana extract, and vanilla. Using an electric mixer, beat in the eggs one at a time until fully combined.

5. Add the dry ingredients to the wet ingredients, and beat on medium-low speed until well incorporated. Add the coconut milk, and continue to mix. Reserve 1 tablespoon of the chocolate chips, then stir in the rest with a wooden spoon.

6. Put the batter in the prepared loaf pan, and sprinkle the reserved chocolate chips on top. Bake for 35 to 40 minutes, or until a toothpick inserted into the center comes out clean.

7. Allow to fully cool on a wire rack before slicing.

8. Store any leftovers in the refrigerator for up to 5 days, or freeze for up to 3 weeks.

Variation Tip: For a more traditional banana bread, leave out the chocolate chips. Or you can kick up the flavor and nutrition by adding in a handful of chopped walnuts.

Per serving: Calories: 254; Total Fat: 21g; Total Carbohydrates: 16g; Net Carbs: 10g; Fiber: 6g; Protein: 6g; Erythritol: 12g
Macros: Fat: 74%; Protein: 9%; Carbs: 17%

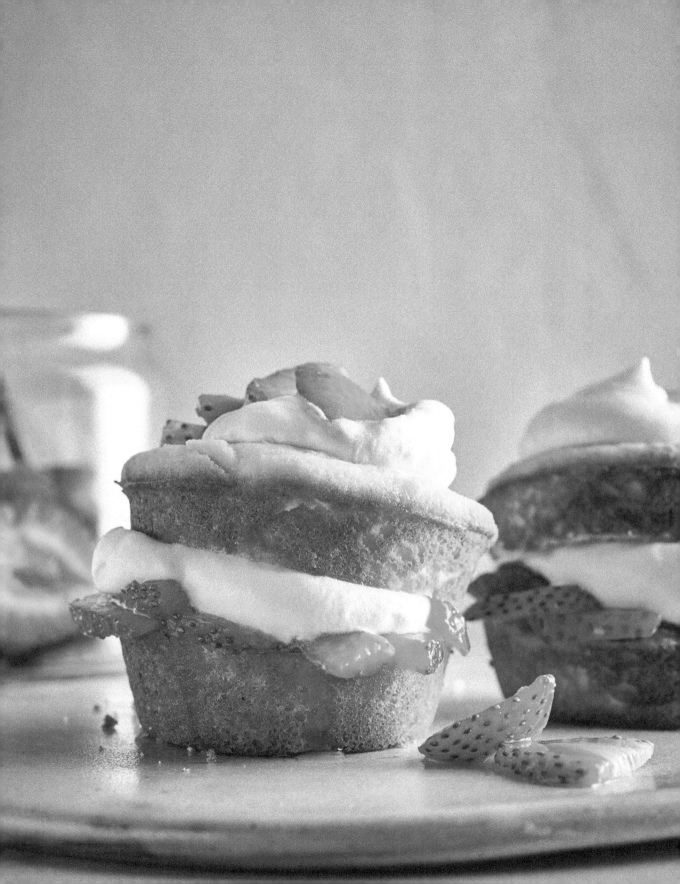

STRAWBERRY SHORTCAKES

MAKES 12 SHORTCAKES / PREP TIME: 15 MINUTES, PLUS MARINATING TIME / COOK TIME: 25 TO 30 MINUTES, PLUS 30 MINUTES TO COOL
EQUIPMENT: 4 MIXING BOWLS, ELECTRIC MIXER, 12-CUP MUFFIN PAN

Strawberry shortcakes have always been a family favorite, and that's why when we went keto, it required a low-carb makeover. For best results, assemble each strawberry shortcake right before serving.

FOR THE SHORTCAKES

4 tablespoons (½ stick) unsalted butter, at room temperature, plus more to grease the pan

¾ cup coconut flour

1 teaspoon baking powder

¼ teaspoon sea salt

¾ cup granulated erythritol–monk fruit blend

4 ounces (about ½ cup) cream cheese, at room temperature

1 teaspoon pure vanilla extract

4 large eggs, at room temperature

¼ cup sour cream

FOR THE STRAWBERRY TOPPING

1 pint fresh strawberries, sliced

2 tablespoons granulated erythritol–monk fruit blend

½ teaspoon freshly squeezed lemon juice

⅛ teaspoon sea salt

FOR THE WHIPPED CREAM

1 cup heavy whipping cream, divided

1 tablespoon cream cheese, at room temperature

2 tablespoons granulated erythritol–monk fruit blend

1 teaspoon pure vanilla extract

TO MAKE THE SHORTCAKES

1. Preheat the oven to 350°F. Generously grease a 12-cup muffin pan with butter.

2. In a medium bowl, combine the coconut flour, baking powder, and salt.

3. In a large bowl, using an electric mixer, beat the erythritol–monk fruit blend, cream cheese, butter, and vanilla until light and fluffy. Add the eggs one at a time, mixing after each addition. Make sure to scrape down the bowl several times. Slowly add the dry ingredients to the wet ingredients while mixing on low speed. Again, make sure to scrape down the sides of the bowl as needed. When fully combined, gently fold in the sour cream, being sure to not overmix.

4. Evenly pour the batter into the muffin pan, overfilling each cup just slightly. Bake for 25 to 30 minutes, or until lightly browned on top and a toothpick inserted into the center comes out clean.

Continued →

5. Allow the shortcakes to cool in the pan for about 10 minutes before removing them. Place them on a wire rack to cool fully, for about 20 minutes.

TO MAKE THE STRAWBERRY TOPPING

1. In a large bowl, combine the sliced strawberries, erythritol–monk fruit blend, lemon juice, and salt.

2. Allow the strawberries to sit at room temperature to macerate for 15 to 30 minutes. This will cause the berries to produce their own sauce.

TO MAKE THE WHIPPED CREAM

1. Chill a large glass or metal mixing bowl in the refrigerator. Using an electric mixer on high speed, beat about ¼ cup of heavy whipping cream with the cream cheese until well combined.

2. Add the remaining ¾ cup of heavy whipping cream, the erythritol–monk fruit blend, and vanilla. Beat on high speed with the electric mixer until soft peaks form and hold their shape.

TO ASSEMBLE THE STRAWBERRY SHORTCAKES

1. Cut each shortcake in half. Place the bottom half of the shortcake on a plate, and spoon on 1 tablespoon of the strawberry topping and 1 tablespoon of the whipped cream.

2. Top with the other half of the shortcake, another tablespoon of whipped cream, and another tablespoon of the strawberry topping.

3. Store any leftovers, without the strawberry topping and the whipped cream, in the refrigerator for up to 5 days, or freeze for up to 3 weeks.

Keep in Mind: The cake batter will be very thick and fluffy. This is the normal texture when using coconut flour exclusively. The thick batter will ensure the muffins don't spread when overfilled.

Per serving: Calories: 216; Total Fat: 18g; Total Carbohydrates: 9g; Net Carbs: 5g; Fiber: 4g; Protein: 5g; Erythritol: 16g
Macros: Fat: 75%; Protein: 9%; Carbs: 16%

CREAM CHEESE POUND CAKE

MAKES 12 SLICES / PREP TIME: 10 MINUTES / COOK TIME: 30 TO 40 MINUTES, PLUS 35 MINUTES TO COOL
EQUIPMENT: 2 MIXING BOWLS, ELECTRIC MIXER, 8-BY-5-INCH LOAF PAN

My Cream Cheese Pound Cake became an instant hit in the keto community when it went viral. It's a rich, moist pound cake that can be enjoyed plain or dressed up with icing or berries.

1¼ cups almond flour, measured
   and sifted
1 teaspoon baking powder
¼ teaspoon sea salt
¾ cup granulated erythritol–monk
   fruit blend

4 tablespoons (½ stick) unsalted butter,
   at room temperature
3½ ounces (about 7 tablespoons)
   cream cheese, at room temperature
1 teaspoon pure vanilla extract
4 large eggs, at room temperature

1. Preheat the oven to 350°F. Line an 8-by-5-inch loaf pan with parchment paper.

2. In a medium bowl, combine the almond flour, baking powder, and salt.

3. In a large bowl, using an electric mixer, cream the erythritol–monk fruit blend with the butter until the mixture is light and fluffy. Add the cream cheese and vanilla, and mix well. Add the eggs one at a time, and mix well after each addition. Add the dry ingredients to the wet ingredients, and mix until fully combined.

4. Pour the batter into the prepared loaf pan. Bake for 30 to 40 minutes, or until golden brown on top. The pound cake is done once a toothpick inserted into the center comes out clean.

5. Allow the cake to cool on a wire rack for 10 minutes before removing from the pan. Then allow to cool for another 25 minutes on a wire rack until fully cooled before slicing.

6. Store any leftovers in the refrigerator for up to 5 days, or freeze for up to 3 weeks.

Variation Tip: Make this into cupcakes! Pour the batter into a lined 12-cup muffin pan, and bake for 20 to 25 minutes.

Per serving: Calories: 154; Total Fat: 14g; Total Carbohydrates: 3g; Net Carbs: 2g;
Fiber: 1g; Protein: 5g; Erythritol: 12g
Macros: Fat: 82%; Protein: 13%; Carbs: 4%

PUMPKIN POUND CAKE

MAKES 12 SLICES / PREP TIME: 10 MINUTES / COOK TIME: 45 TO 50 MINUTES, PLUS 35 MINUTES TO COOL
EQUIPMENT: 3 MIXING BOWLS, ELECTRIC MIXER, 9-BY-5-INCH LOAF PAN

If there is one dessert you will want to make all through the fall, it's this pumpkin pound cake. The cake is bursting with spices and is a flavorful, seasonal treat. I have also included an optional vanilla icing that further elevates the cake, making it one you'll be proud to share during the winter holidays.

FOR THE POUND CAKE
1½ cups finely milled almond flour, measured and sifted
1½ tablespoons ground cinnamon
1½ teaspoons ground ginger
1½ teaspoons pumpkin pie spice
1½ teaspoons baking powder
½ teaspoon ground nutmeg
¼ teaspoon ground allspice
⅛ teaspoon ground cloves
¼ teaspoon sea salt
¾ cup granulated erythritol–monk fruit blend
8 tablespoons (1 stick) unsalted butter, at room temperature

¼ cup brown or golden granulated erythritol–monk fruit blend
4 ounces (about ½ cup) cream cheese, at room temperature
1 teaspoon pure vanilla extract
½ cup canned pumpkin purée
3 large eggs, at room temperature

FOR THE ICING
½ cup confectioners' erythritol–monk fruit blend
3 to 4 tablespoons heavy whipping cream, plus more as needed
½ teaspoon pure vanilla extract

TO MAKE THE POUND CAKE

1. Preheat the oven to 350°F. Line a 9-by-5-inch loaf pan with parchment paper.

2. In a medium bowl, combine the almond flour, cinnamon, ginger, pumpkin pie spice, baking powder, nutmeg, allspice, cloves, and salt.

3. In a large bowl, using an electric mixer, cream the erythritol–monk fruit blend, butter, and brown erythritol–monk fruit blend until the mixture is light and fluffy and well incorporated. Add the cream cheese and vanilla, and mix well. Add the pumpkin purée, and mix until just incorporated.

4. Alternate adding the eggs one at a time with the dry ingredients, and mix thoroughly after each addition. Scrape down the sides of the bowl periodically.

5. Pour the batter into the prepared pan. Bake for 45 to 50 minutes, or until golden brown on top. The pound cake is done when a toothpick inserted into the center comes out clean.

6. Allow to cool on a wire rack for 10 minutes before removing the cake from the pan. Then allow to cool for another 25 minutes on a wire rack until fully cooled before icing.

TO MAKE THE ICING AND FINISH THE CAKE

1. In a small bowl, put the confectioners' erythritol–monk fruit blend, and whisk in the heavy whipping cream and vanilla, making sure to fully incorporate the mixture. Add more heavy whipping cream if the icing is too thick; it should be runny enough to drizzle.

2. Once the pound cake has fully cooled, drizzle on the icing, and serve.

3. Store any leftovers in the refrigerator for up to 5 days, or freeze for up to 3 weeks.

Variation Tip: You can also bake this cake in a large Bundt pan for a stunning presentation. Simply double the recipe, and bake for about 60 to 70 minutes. Allow the cake to cool in the pan on a wire rack for about 10 minutes before taking it out of the pan. Then place the cake on the wire rack for another 25 minutes to fully cool before icing or slicing.

Per serving: Calories: 221; Total Fat: 21g; Total Carbohydrates: 6g; Net Carbs: 3g; Fiber: 3g; Protein: 6g; Erythritol: 22g
Macros: Fat: 86%; Protein: 11%; Carbs: 3%

RASPBERRY-LEMON POUND CAKE

MAKES 10 SLICES / PREP TIME: 10 MINUTES / COOK TIME: 35 TO 40 MINUTES, PLUS 30 TO 35 MINUTES TO COOL
EQUIPMENT: 3 MIXING BOWLS, ELECTRIC MIXER, 9-BY-5-INCH LOAF PAN

Full of bright, cheery raspberries, this easy keto dessert is sure to become a favorite. With just a few ingredients, you can enjoy a pound cake that will have you thinking you're cheating. I love how the sweetness of the cream cheese pairs well with the tartness of the berries. And because I can't leave good enough alone, this recipe also includes a vanilla glaze, which adds yet another layer of flavor.

FOR THE POUND CAKE
Coconut oil, for greasing the pan
1¼ cups finely milled almond flour, measured and sifted
1¼ teaspoons baking powder
¼ teaspoon sea salt
4 ounces (about ½ cup) cream cheese, at room temperature
½ cup granulated erythritol–monk fruit blend
4 tablespoons (½ stick) unsalted butter, at room temperature

2 teaspoons grated lemon zest
1 teaspoon liquid lemon extract
4 large eggs, at room temperature
1 cup fresh or frozen whole raspberries

FOR THE VANILLA GLAZE
½ cup confectioners' erythritol–monk fruit blend
2 to 3 tablespoons heavy whipping cream
½ teaspoon pure vanilla extract

TO MAKE THE POUND CAKE

1. Preheat the oven to 350°F. Lightly grease a 9-by-5-inch loaf pan with coconut oil.

2. In a medium bowl, combine the almond flour, baking powder, and salt.

3. In a large bowl, using an electric mixer on medium speed, cream the cream cheese, erythritol–monk fruit blend, butter, lemon zest, and lemon extract until light and fluffy. Scrape down the sides of the bowl with a spatula. Add the eggs one at a time, and mix on medium speed after each addition until the eggs are blended. Scrape down the sides of the bowl each time. Add the dry ingredients to the wet batter, beating on low speed until well incorporated.

4. Reserving 2 tablespoons, gently fold the raspberries into the batter with a rubber spatula. Spread the mixture in the prepared loaf pan, and top with the reserved raspberries, pressing them into the batter.

5. Bake the loaf for 35 to 40 minutes, or until the top springs back to the touch and a toothpick inserted into the center comes out clean.

6. Allow the pound cake to cool in the pan for about 15 minutes before unmolding. Then allow to cool on a wire rack for another 15 to 20 minutes before icing.

TO MAKE THE VANILLA GLAZE AND FINISH THE CAKE

1. Combine the confectioners' erythritol–monk fruit blend, 2 tablespoons heavy whipping cream, and vanilla. Add another tablespoon of heavy whipping cream if the glaze is too thick.

2. Drizzle over the pound cake once it's cooled.

3. Store any leftovers in the refrigerator for up to 5 days, or freeze for up to 3 weeks.

Variation Tip: If you're unable to get raspberries or want to try a different flavor, you can substitute them with fresh or frozen blueberries or blackberries.

Per serving: Calories: 206; Total Fat: 19g; Total Carbohydrates: 5g; Net Carbs: 3g; Fiber: 2g; Protein: 7g; Erythritol: 17g
Macros: Fat: 83%; Protein: 14%; Carbs: 3%

LEMON CURD LAYER CAKE

MAKES 12 SLICES / PREP TIME: 15 MINUTES / COOK TIME: 35 TO 40 MINUTES, PLUS 40 MINUTES TO COOL
EQUIPMENT: 2 MIXING BOWLS, ELECTRIC MIXER, MEDIUM SAUCEPAN, 2 (9-INCH) CAKE PANS

This lemon curd layer cake is for lemon lovers. Bursting with lusciously sweet and tart flavor, it features layers of moist, lemony cake and velvety smooth lemon curd. Because of its richness, it requires no frosting. Make the curd while the cakes are baking, so it has plenty of time to chill in the refrigerator.

FOR THE LEMON CURD

5 tablespoons unsalted butter

8 large egg yolks, at room temperature

1 cup granulated erythritol–monk fruit blend

1 cup freshly squeezed lemon juice

1 tablespoon grated lemon zest

½ teaspoon lemon extract

¼ teaspoon sea salt

FOR THE CAKE

4 tablespoons (½ stick) unsalted butter, softened, plus more to grease the pans

4 ounces (about ½ cup) cream cheese, softened

1 cup granulated erythritol–monk fruit blend

4 large eggs, at room temperature

1¼ cups finely milled almond flour, measured and sifted

1 teaspoon baking powder

1 teaspoon grated lemon zest

¼ teaspoon sea salt

3 tablespoons freshly squeezed lemon juice

1 teaspoon lemon extract

TO MAKE THE LEMON CURD

1. Fill a saucepan two-thirds full with simmering water, then set a heat-proof bowl above it and use that to melt the butter. Add the egg yolks one at a time, whisking quickly to incorporate each one. While continuing to whisk, add the erythritol–monk fruit blend, lemon juice, lemon zest, lemon extract, and salt.

2. Mix until all the ingredients are combined and the lemon curd thickens. This will take anywhere from 5 to 7 minutes.

3. If you want, you can push the curd through a fine-mesh sieve to remove the lemon zest and to ensure that it's velvety smooth.

4. Put the bowl of lemon curd in the refrigerator with plastic wrap on the surface of the curd, so a crust does not form on top.

TO MAKE THE CAKE

1. Preheat the oven 350°F. Grease 2 (9-inch) baking pans with butter.

2. In a large bowl, using an electric mixer on high speed cream the butter and cream cheese until light and fluffy. While mixing, add the erythritol–monk fruit blend.

3. Add the eggs one at a time, mixing well after each addition. Stir in the almond flour, baking powder, lemon zest, and salt, and mix well. Add the lemon juice and lemon extract, and beat until the batter is fully mixed.

4. Pour the batter evenly into the 2 cake pans, and bake for 35 to 40 minutes, or until a toothpick inserted into the center comes out clean.

5. Allow the cakes to cool in their pans for 10 minutes, then remove them from their pans. Place the cakes on a wire rack, and allow to cool for another 30 minutes until fully cooled.

TO ASSEMBLE THE CAKE

1. Put one of the cakes on a cake stand or flat plate, and spread half the lemon curd on top.

2. Carefully place the second cake on top, and spread the rest of the lemon curd on top.

3. Store any leftovers in the refrigerator for up to 5 days, or freeze for up to 3 weeks.

Variation Tip: Grate a little more lemon zest, and use it to decorate the top of the cake, along with some fresh raspberries, for a pop of color and extra flavor.

Per serving: Calories: 242; Total Fat: 22g; Total Carbohydrates: 6g; Net Carbs: 5g; Fiber: 1g; Protein: 7g; Erythritol: 32g
Macros: Fat: 82%; Protein: 12%; Carbs: 6%

MEASUREMENT CONVERSIONS

Volume Equivalents (Liquid)

US Standard	US Standard (ounces)	Metric (approximate)
2 tablespoons	1 fl. oz.	30 mL
¼ cup	2 fl. oz.	60 mL
½ cup	4 fl. oz.	120 mL
1 cup	8 fl. oz.	240 mL
1½ cups	12 fl. oz.	355 mL
2 cups or 1 pint	16 fl. oz.	475 mL
4 cups or 1 quart	32 fl. oz.	1 L
1 gallon	128 fl. oz.	4 L

Oven Temperatures

Fahrenheit (F)	Celsius (C) (approximate)
250°F	120°C
300°F	150°C
325°F	165°C
350°F	180°C
375°F	190°C
400°F	200°C
425°F	220°C
450°F	230°C

Volume Equivalents (Dry)

US Standard	Metric (approximate)
⅛ teaspoon	0.5 mL
¼ teaspoon	1 mL
½ teaspoon	2 mL
¾ teaspoon	4 mL
1 teaspoon	5 mL
1 tablespoon	15 mL
¼ cup	59 mL
⅓ cup	79 mL
½ cup	118 mL
⅔ cup	156 mL
¾ cup	177 mL
1 cup	235 mL
2 cups or 1 pint	475 mL
3 cups	700 mL
4 cups or 1 quart	1 L

Weight Equivalents

US Standard	Metric (approximate)
½ ounce	15 g
1 ounce	30 g
2 ounces	60 g
4 ounces	115 g
8 ounces	225 g
12 ounces	340 g
16 ounces or 1 pound	455 g

RESOURCES

INFORMATIONAL RESOURCES

Ketogenic

Ketogenic.com

A trusted resource for the keto community that offers quality education and information on the ketogenic diet. The site includes articles, tips, recipes, and tools from top thought leaders and doctors.

Keto Calculator

PerfectKeto.com/keto-macro-calculator/

An easy, free ketogenic macro calculator that lets you calculate your personal keto macros in minutes. It will help you find the exact amount of carbs, fat, and protein you need to reach your goal weight using the ketogenic diet.

Dr. Eric Berg

www.DrBerg.com

www.youtube.com/watch?v=vMZfyEy_jpl

Dr. Berg is one of the top ketogenic diet experts. He shares vital information on how to properly do the diet to see results. He is a health educator who specializes in weight loss through nutritional and natural methods by combining the keto diet with intermittent fasting.

Dr. Eric Westman

www.facebook.com/pages/category/Doctor/Dr-Eric-Westman-127133981830/

Dr. Westman is a renowned expert in low-carb diets, diabetes and obesity, and insulin resistance. He is an associate professor of medicine at Duke University Health System and director of the Duke Lifestyle Medicine Clinic.

The Ketogenic Bible, The Authoritative Guide to Ketosis

By Dr. Jacob Wilson and Ryan Lowery, Ph.D. (Victory Belt Publishing, 2017)

This book takes a comprehensive look at the keto diet and fat-burning state of ketosis. It has the most up-to-date information on how the keto diet affects the body. Their approach is based on a wide range of scientific research, including the research they are doing at their own Applied Science and Performance Institute.

ONLINE STORES

Anthony's Goods

www.AnthonysGoods.com

A great place to buy almond flour, coconut flour, and other alternatives to wheat flour, as well as sugar substitutes.

Bob's Red Mill

www.BobsRedMill.com

Bob's makes a lot of alternative flours. You can find Bob's Red Mill products in many supermarkets, as well as on their website.

Lakanto Monk Fruit Sweeteners

www.Lakanto.com

Erythritol–monk fruit is my go-to choice for sweeteners. Lakanto sources all their monk fruit in the highlands of Asia, a pristine area, and using environmental methods.

NOW Foods

www.NowFoods.com

NOW makes a variety of flours, sweeteners, binders, and nut and seed products, including golden flax meal. Their website includes a section just for keto diets.

OOOFlavors

www.OOOFlavors.com

OOOFlavors makes delicious flavor extracts, monk fruit–based sweeteners, and sugar-free syrups.

BRICK AND MORTAR STORES

Trader Joe's

Trader Joe's is a great neighborhood grocery store with stores nationwide. It is a great place to find organic produce and products at reasonable prices.

Whole Foods Market

Whole Foods sells natural and organic foods and has a strong emphasis on sustainable agriculture. Amazon Prime Members who have stores near them get free two-hour delivery.

RECIPE INDEX

INDEX

ACKNOWLEDGMENTS

I'll start by thanking my husband, Randy, who makes me feel I can do anything. Love, I am forever grateful that you agreed to do the keto diet together with me. You've tested every single one of my recipes, even the ones that never made the cut and landed in the trash. Randy, you may not have written this book, but it is as much yours as mine. Without you, there would be no FITTOSERVE and indeed no recipes to speak of.

The tireless work of my daughter, Michelle, is what made this book possible. She was part of the entire process, from helping me decide what recipes to include to tasting and assisting me in formatting. Thank you so very much, Cuchita, for your support and for keeping me sane in the process. Thank you to my son, Matthew, for your humor and for keeping me smiling through the whole writing process. Peter, my son-in-love, thank you for using your education in statistics to assist me in recipe development. And for putting up with the constant interruptions as I leaned on Michelle to help me see the book through to completion.

Creating recipes is a messy endeavor with piles of dishes that no one wants to tackle, so immense thanks to Paul, my brother, for rolling up your sleeves and taking care of the cleanup. Thank you to my little sis, Lisa, for encouraging me and for taking care of Mom when pressing deadlines made it impossible for me to be as present as I wanted to be. You have a way of supporting the entire family like no one else.

Mami, thank you for showing me how to cook with love and for demonstrating generosity and kindness like the true angel you are. You will forever be my example of a Proverbs 31 woman. Papi, you are the true artist in the family, and I just took some of your heart to express myself in the recipes here. Thank you for always encouraging me to think outside the box and to explore every angle.

To Martha Avila, my mentor and close friend, thank you for faithfully supporting me through some of my darkest challenges and for championing my idea to start FITTOSERVE. Special thanks to my pastors, Ricky and Yvette Gallinar, who had a front seat to my health transformation and believed with our family when hope seemed lost.

You fully embraced the vision of FITTOSERVE, and your prophetic words spoke this book into existence.

I am blessed by a large extended and church family that has for years faithfully supported me. I hope this book serves to encourage you to see the goodness of our God in a palpable manner.

This book is for my blog followers. Every recipe you shared and picture you sent me of your creations has served as a vehicle to force me to grow. This book exists because of you.

Last but certainly not least, special thanks to Ada Fung, my editor, and to everyone at Callisto Media who worked to make this book a reality.

ABOUT THE AUTHOR

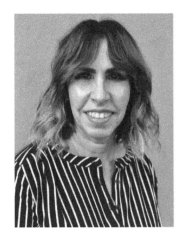

Hilda Solares holds a bachelor of arts degree in theology from the Latin University of Theology. She has worked in a variety of positions in education, with close to 30 years of experience. Hilda also has an extensive ministry background with more than 25 years of service. In 2014, she founded Fit To Serve Group, a church community group that combines the Christian faith with a low-carb keto diet. Hilda shares her ketogenic recipes on her blog, FitToServeGroup.com. The group is where she and her husband, Randy Solares, teach the community how to combine biblical principles with healthy eating habits for greater health and wellness. Her life work aims to encourage people to eat well and feel well to be able to serve well.

CPSIA information can be obtained
at www.ICGtesting.com
Printed in the USA
LVHW012119061219
639669LV00005B/9/P